REIKI: A SPIRITUAL DOORWAY

TO NATURAL HEALING

Eileen Curteis

*To Krysta,
a warm and
wonderful soul.
God's love,
blessing and
healing be
with you.
Sister Eileen*

Printed in Victoria, Canada

Cover Photo: Carol Porteous-Crawford
Text Drawings: Eileen Curteis

Some of these poems and prose pieces have appeared in the following books, journals and newspapers: *Prairie Messenger, paperplates, L'Antenne, Grail, Canadian Woman Studies, Wind Daughter, Poetry and Spiritual Practice.*

ACKNOWLEDGEMENTS:
I would like to thank Sue Hansen for producing the CD at the back of this book. Because of Sue's giftedness as a composer, musical arranger and vocalist, she has enhanced my work by setting a number of my poems to music. Karen S. Williamson, the composer for two of the songs and the pianist who provided the background music for my poetry has also enriched my book. Special thanks to Carol-Porteous Crawford for her encouragement and editing of this book, and to Sheila Hughes, ssa, for her computer skills and great generosity in putting this manuscipt together.

Published in conjunction with The Sisters of Saint Ann and Trafford Publishing.

A cataloguing record for this book that includes the U.S. Library of Congress Classification number, the Library of Congress Call number and the Dewey Decimal cataloguing code is available from the National Library of Canada. The complete cataloguing record can be obtained from the National Library's online database at: www.nlc-bnc.ca/amicus/index-e.html
ISBN 1-4120-2165-0

TRAFFORD

This book was published *on-demand* in cooperation with Trafford Publishing.
On-demand publishing is a unique process and service of making a book available for retail sale to the public taking advantage of on-demand manufacturing and Internet marketing.
On-demand publishing includes promotions, retail sales, manufacturing, order fulfilment, accounting and collecting royalties on behalf of the author.

Suite 6E, 2333 Government St., Victoria, B.C. V8T 4P4, CANADA

Phone	250-383-6864	Toll-free	1-888-232-4444 (Canada & US)
Fax	250-383-6804	E-mail	sales@trafford.com
Web site	www.trafford.com	TRAFFORD PUBLISHING IS A DIVISION OF TRAFFORD HOLDINGS LTD.	
Trafford Catalogue #03-2714		www.trafford.com/robots/03-2714.html	

10   9   8   7   6   5   4   3   2

DEDICATION

"We have the power to let the current pass through
us to produce the light of the world.
. . . Mother Teresa

For my family, my friends
and all those in the Reiki community
who have helped me tap into the
wondrous healing Energy
of God with us.

CONTENTS

FOREWORD

How can anyone begin to write a story as complex as mine? This was the question I asked myself five years ago when a number of people suggested my healing journey needed to be told and shared.

As a writer, I know that timing is important and that one cannot force the hand of the Spirit until the season is right and the gift is given. Seven years ago, the seed was planted by a beautiful woman called Carole who was sent into my life quite unexpectedly. She is one of God's modern day prophets who knew all about my writing and how the plan would unfold. Before she came, I had decided to self publish because of the repeated rejection of my work by secular companies but she insisted that this was not the route to go. Through her guidance, I was led to a Victoria publisher, Richard, whose spirituality resonated with mine. What transpired seemed to be of divine origin and two of my books were published through him. Now, six years later, the Sisters of Saint Ann are publishing my work, honouring the gift that I bring.

When I first met Carole, seven years ago, she asked me about my unpublished manuscripts hidden in my cupboard. I was shocked to think she would have this kind of knowledge. I showed her the manuscripts written back in 1966. As she looked through them, she said, "You will select poems from them and your writing style will change." I had no idea how this could come to pass but in the spring of March, 2001, I met a gifted composer, Karen Williamson, from Sequim, Washington, who felt called to set my work to music. Thirty-five years prior, some of my close friends had said, "Your poems are lovely. They should be set to music." I remember the initial thrill, feeling privileged to think that God might be picking me, along with others, to deliver a message I longed to share. At the time, my wings weren't ready but now, thirty-five years later with Karen's coming, my heart and soul have taken flight.

As I returned to the original poems in the manuscript, I

was inspired to bring them to completion. The words came quickly and the music followed. Karen was like another Beethoven. The music flooded into her, non-stop night and day until she had completed twenty compositions. Simultaneously, the musicians were drawn together to bring about the full orchestration of Karen's gift. *Dance of the Mystic Healer,* has now taken on a life of its own. The book of healing poems, sketches and photography, with myself reciting the poems on CD came first. Then, came a second CD with my poems being sung and accompanied by gifted musicians. They are passionate Love songs inspiring people to find the Divine in themselves, in others and in the whole of cosmic Creation. Our sole purpose in putting out the work was to give glory to God and bring healing into the lives of those it would touch.

As early as 1966, my poetry and art were already hinting at the demanding healing passage I would one day undergo. One of my later poems describes the Journey succinctly.

TOUGH AS STEEL

A butterfly of sorts
she comes stomping
out of her frail delicate wings.
Frost bitten in winter
she grows soft petals
tough as steel.

Rains come,
winds blow,
blizzards fall,
there is nothing
she can't withstand.

Like pinched skin
or burnt grass
in a stubby field
hardship
is something she walks through.

My earlier manuscripts were prophetically telling the story and the reason I feel the work was never published was because I had not gone through the healing that was required. In 1977, sketches were given to complement the prose poems. As these visions appeared on paper, I felt elated, treasuring them in my heart, intuitively knowing that one day my healing would occur.

Today, it is with integrity I tell my story and, as Carole predicted, I have selected poems and sketches that will help convey the message. Added to this is the music of Karen and Sue that makes for a more elated rendering of the story.

In my long space of waiting, I now understand, it was Sue Hansen's extraordinary voice that was needed to complete what I have so earnestly felt called to share. Sue's unexpected arrival and journeying with me appears in the epilogue of my book.

What is important to note is that the spirituality in this book is my spirituality, rooted in Scripture and flowing from the tradition of the mystics. My road would seem to be that of the mystic, one who knows God by personal intervention. My story is based on a personal journey and a personal interpretation of circumstances and happenings in a conscious faith context. In sharing this experience, it is my hope that others will benefit spiritually from it and will be empowered to pursue their own healing journeys.

Why I should have been led through an eastern door to find the missing tool of my healing, God alone knows. Perhaps it is to say to the churches and western medicine, there's a complementary form of healing out there that grass roots people know about. I'm convinced the proverb Jesus quotes, "Physician, heal yourself," will be the new medicine of the future as each of us takes responsibility to search out root issues as to why we are ill. This is not to put a damper on western medicine because it does have its place but rather it is to challenge a system that lacks answers for some of the most critical problems of our day. I am grateful that I fit into the area called critical because had I not grown disillusioned with a medical system that was unable to help me, I would not now be in the most wondrous healing passage of my life.

In addressing complementary healing, I am just one of the many grains of sand on a beach, feeling called to have my voice be heard. In the telling of my story, I would like to impart to you, how Reiki, gift of God, became an avenue of healing for me and many others. It may be a path you choose to follow.

As we move through the new millennium, I believe that we are going to explore the frontiers of healing in a whole new way and that Reiki is just one of them. I believe holistic healing will be one of the greatest adventures of our century and for those of us who have the courage to embark on it, we will each in our turn be trail blazers who leave a legacy for the generations to come. It is together in community we make our journey.

MY STORY

My story is one of celebration, hope, joy, recovery. There's nothing of blame in it and, yet, inherent in my destiny is a severity I was meant to undergo in order to arrive at the fullness of my healing.

You might call me a desert traveller who found herself parched enough to go in search of an oasis because truly, that's been the story of my life.

If I said to you, "I chose to become sick in order to become well," you most probably would say, "What a ridiculous thing to do." And yet, after sixty-one years of travelling I know I am as sane as anyone, and that the Waters I have drunk from have brought me the restoration I went in search of.

Since the medical world had no answers for a journey like mine, I chose a complementary route of healing and breakthrough that brought me the wholeness and exhilaration I longed for.

This is my story, and most probably the story of countless others, the specifics different, but the journey similar.

Come with me, now, as I share the story of a girl called "Small" who will one day grow into a strong, beautiful woman aware of her Divine destiny to heal and be healed.

THE WOUNDED GIRL

Age four, a small girl falls down on the road. Her right knee splits. She goes to the doctor who puts stitches in her knee. She's a brave girl and tries not to cry. She's an awkward girl and she keeps falling. Every time she falls her knee splits and she goes through the same procedure. Finally, her parents take her to Vancouver where there is supposed to be a famous bandage that will be put on her knee and prevent it from splitting. She returns to Victoria, an ecstatic little girl who isn't afraid to fall anymore. She goes running down hill to the grocery store. She falls on her right knee and feels a wet something trickling down. It's red and messy and the bandage won't stop it. She bellows at her parents and tells them she doesn't want to go to the doctor this time. It doesn't make any difference, the louder she bellows they still insist on taking her. She resents her parents. Simultaneously, "I hate the doctor" syndrome begins. She keeps falling until she makes a deliberate choice around age seven not to fall anymore. At this time, the "over cautious" syndrome begins. She can still remember the first time she ran in a school race so far behind the others, she lost sight of them. Feeling like a total failure was a new experience for her. From then on, in sports and gym, she was like a turtle holding her feet in and going nowhere fast. Nobody, you can be sure, wanted her on their team. Unbeknown to her, the fear of falling and the physical tightening of her muscles would eventually lead to an imprisoned body that would force her to look at life in a new way.

Age five, she sees her parents in an angry mood, expressing themselves in a way that is healthy, but horrifying to a youngster her age. Terrified by the ugliness of their faces, she makes a deliberate choice never to be like them, a pattern that persists long into adult life. It's the "nice girl never gets angry" syndrome. Coupled with this, is the good little bad little girl theory she learned in church or at catechism. Even a slight irritation is sinful for her. Little did she realize that her recurring depressions from childhood were intricately connected with her inability to get angry. She gave her power away at such an early age and never regained it until her thirty ninth year when she was visited by a horrific breakdown, the beginning of her breakthrough.

Age six, the "ugly girl" syndrome begins where children and parents make fun of her size. The first day on her way to school a parent says, "She's no more than three! What's she doing at school?" There's really nothing wrong with this little girl but her hypersensitive nature reads into this statement "tiny is ugly." All through her school years, children, teachers, and people make fun of her size. In her adult life, the sarcasm continues, some people inferring she didn't make it to womanhood and she stupidly believes them. In a poem called, "Small's World", she tells us what it's like to live this way.

SMALL'S WORLD
I
Small
is a little girl
who lived sometime
before the war was over
but for Small
the war was never over.
It was just beginning.
One day
Small told her friend:
"When war comes
do not remove these hornets
from my song birds
in the trenches
but let me hear in them
the thunder of my own bullets.
Then teach me courage
how to die
kissing the lips of my toad."
II
Small starts out early
but in the big world
Small gets crushed easily.

Small hates death.
Small hates life.
Small hates everything.
Small is never big.
Small is always small.
Death is small
as small as Small.

III

Small goes to school.
Small hurts.
Small hides.
Small goes into a corner.
Small sees no one.
No one sees Small.
Small is small,
and death is small,
as small as Small.

IV

It's dark
in Small's world.
Everything is dark.
The food is dark.
The bed is dark.
Small fears the dark!
Small fears everything!

V

Small smiles.
Small sings.
But Small doesn't know
why she does these things.
Small you see
can see no sky,
Small you see
only wants to die.

VI

Small never grows big.
But big grows small.
Small pushes her way
up the stairs

and falls less often
when she gets there.
At the top
Small changes.
Small likes to change.
Small sees
things differently.

VII

In the morning
Small puts seeds
on the window.
Birds come
and she sees them.
At night
she closes the door
and it is light
in her room.
People come
and she lets them in.
Small is growing big.

VIII

Small likes to be big.
But Small
is never too big.
Small likes people.
People like Small.
Small goes out.
Small comes in.
Small
is unafraid of Small.

From an early age, her story gets complicated. Her size embarrasses her and she tenses up her buttock muscles trying to make herself taller. When she sits in her desk at school, when she goes to church to pray, when she talks to anyone bigger than she is, she tenses up her muscles. It's an automatic nerve response. She's like a baby giraffe, twelve hours a day, three hundred sixty five days a year, trying to stretch her neck just one inch taller. Nobody suspects her tactics and, so, in her teenage years it's no wonder she's in chronic pain. Walking is difficult, dancing unbearable.

Age fifteen, her pain gets recognized. She's in hospital for severe scoliosis. She feels ecstatic as she did at age four. Back specialists are going to help her. Everything will be fine. The day for diagnosis comes. Two doctors examine her. She stands there, stripped and naked, ashamed that she doesn't have any breasts. The doctors are cold, aloof. One of them traces his finger down her back and says, "If your spine had developed properly you would be three inches taller. If we do surgery, you'll be paralyzed. The physiotherapist will show you some exercises that you need to do everyday of your life. We'll also set you up with a traction board you can use when you come home from school. There's nothing more we can do for you so learn to live with your pain." Her sciatica is killing her. She's tensing her body tighter than ever. She's cringing from the inside out. She says to herself, "I'll never complain again. I'll live with this pain. I'll keep my mouth shut." She's thinking to herself, I don't ever want to go near a doctor's office again. It's too devastating in there. I'll keep my mouth shut. And, so, the "chronic pain shut your mouth" syndrome is there to stay. Her spirituality supports this too. "Pick up your cross and follow me." She does it cheerfully because she's a brave girl who knows how to turn the other cheek.

After her sojourn in hospital, she undergoes chiropractic treatments which are intended to help her. They have the opposite effect. She's not ready for this aggressive kind of male energy. Her body stiffens like a board, freezes with each onslaught of physical adjustment. It might as well be a lion pouncing on her, so terrorized is she by these treatments. Her body is small and bruises easily. She hides the welts but in private looks at them and knows they are there. Finally, after several treatments, the chiropractor says he can't help her. She's delighted, feeling free and liberated but the negativity stays with her. Any time a male person approaches her it triggers a kind of fear over which she has no control. She knows from experience male energy can hurt her and from now on wants to avoid it. She builds walls, high ones, that nobody can climb over or through.

Most of her negative patterns begin at age six. She doesn't have a voice of her own so if a person says jump through a hoop, she jumps through a hoop. She's a timid girl trying to please everyone, her mother, her father, her teacher, her brother. She's wearing so many different hats and none of them fit. She's already learned to smile and be happy but inside she's a bundle of nerves and nerves don't learn well at school. Her dad's a principal, a genius, so she's told. People have high expectations for the principal's daughter. She pretends to be learning but she's taking in nothing. She's caught up in fear and her brain doesn't function well. Can't think, can't talk, can't remember. She's in a fog the whole time she's at school, worse yet at university. She hates tests, and puts answers down like a dumb parrot, forgetting everything she ever learned. Wherever she goes, it's the "stupid kid" syndrome that follows her. Without a voice she can't tell anyone what's happening, not even her parents or the children on the playground. She's a shy girl who doesn't fit into groups, a social misfit, a loner who's terrified the big kids are going to get her when she walks home from school.

When she gets home she likes it because it's safe in her house. Her mother loves her, protects her. She's a good mother who would never let anybody harm her daughter. It's the "mother smother" syndrome she buys into. She doesn't need a voice because her mother has it for her. She loves her dad. He's a kind, clever, humourous man and she wants to be like him but she knows she will never be like him because she doesn't function well at school.

Years later, when the breakthrough comes, she begins to function well and describes her new found freedom in a poem entitled, "I Found My Poppies Outside The System."

I FOUND MY POPPIES OUTSIDE THE SYSTEM

I am a winter bird
that has no place
to lay its head.
I am winter all over
with a song in my heart
and no one to hear.
I sit on people's windows
pecking
at their closed-inness.
I sing
far beyond my strength
for the day
when they shall hear
and I will be gone.

Migrating south
I could be as present as your finger is
or as anonymous as my name has become.
A stranger at school today
nobody sees
the cavity called loneliness
in the desk where I sit.
Like a sliver of wood
I am too small
to be seen by anyone.
I have gone to this school
for twelve years now,
but I am too small
to be seen by anyone.

At university
I play the game
called funeral.
Nobody attends the ceremony.
Only my books do.
Years later,
like sunshine

spurting out
from under the closed lid
of a coffin,
I kiss that stupid kid
in a wastebasket
better.

I'm a degreed person
who found her poppies
outside the system.

Another kind of school she attends are catechism classes on Saturday or Sunday, but sometimes she doesn't like what she hears. She has her own ideas about God. Where they come from, she's not quite sure, but she thinks she knows God better than some of the things she's being taught. She stumbles through prayers at catechism school but at home she talks to God like a friend. She's a spiritual girl who loves God from the beginning. She could be knocked over by a car or tumble down a hill and still she'd know God loves her. That's the kind of faith she has. She's a gentle girl with a strong, sturdy spirit. Whenever things go wrong, which is most of the time, she turns to God as the one companion who will never let her down. She identifies with Jesus, the lamb of God, and chooses to be as gentle as He was. It's a passive kind of spirituality, good for now, but that will one day do damage to her.

Many devastating things happen to her as a young girl. By the time she matures into puberty, her negative patterns have already been well established and she is totally out of touch with her feelings. Everything that hurts or causes pain, she swallows and represses it in her body. She's a sick girl to whom the experience of shut down comes early but nobody reads the signs because of the happy mask she wears. One doctor in her teenage years recognizes her disfigurement and asks, "Did you have rickets when you were little?" Her body cringes and says, "I don't think so. What's that?" On finding out what's that, her body cringes some more and the ugly duckling wraps its arms around her as she leaves the office more ashamed than when she went in. She tells her mother about the experience and wishes she hadn't. Her mother gets angry and says she was a well fed little girl. The cement wall grows bigger than ever. Ugly is in. Ugly is there to stay.

For years and years, she struggles with a hardship called insomnia better known as depression but she doesn't know it's depression. She hates going to bed at night, hates the dark, hates not being able to sleep. She wonders how she can drag herself to school the next day but drags herself she does. As listless as she is, she's long suffering and determined to make a success of her life, to get through the school system without it totally destroying her. Were it not for her morals and the immense love she has for God, she would have ended it long before now. She knows that.

THE SEARCHING WOMAN

Age nineteen, she enters religious life and asks herself, "How come my soul is on fire with love for God? Where did this passion come from?" She knows it's not a figment of her imagination. She feels the pulse of her heart and she knows it's for real. A Presence invades her, overtakes her. What's happening is ethereal, mystical. You won't find it in the scientific data of our age because nothing like this gets recorded. She's entered a new plane of being and will never return to the old, so she thinks. She lives this way for eight years, totally positive and driven by spiritual energy. Wherever she goes, she's in love with God, herself, people, planet earth. She tells us about her passion for life in the following poem.

FIRE WOMAN

Blessed be the rose
that falls once too often
she shall see God.
Blessed be her body, the scarecrow,
that brings forth life from the tomb.
She shall be the mother of many.
Blessed be her spirit.
She shall bring forth stars from a stone
and no one shall go hungry from her.
Blessed be the air that floats in
at her window.
It shall hoist her up like a sail.
Blessed be the River that springs up
like a faucet in her.
It shall gush forth like a stream.
Blessed the woman, who warms her feet
on the coals of this Fire,
she shall be heated from within!

She knows all about giving and nothing about boundaries.

Age twenty-seven, she makes a crash landing. Her whole body is wired, out of balance. It's like electrical currents going through her every fifteen minutes. It's so jarring she can hardly bear it. She's never heard of a nervous breakdown but this is what she's going through. Can't eat, can't sleep. Her body's killing her. This time she thinks she's dying. She ends up in hospital for two weeks. All the scientific tests that the medical world knows are administered. Diagnosis, "physically well, nothing wrong". In the poem, "The Girl Called Worry", she addresses the medical world's inability to understand what is happening to her.

THE GIRL CALLED WORRY

Locked in a cupboard
hiding on a shelf
Worry is a fidgety girl
who can't do things right.

In the morning she dresses herself
but the clothes don't fit.
Worry is slim. Worry is fat.
Worry is never what she wants to be.

With feet too big for her
Worry goes shopping
and the groceries tumble.
Worry trips. Worry falls.
Worry never goes anywhere
without breaking things.

At school
Worry is the timid little goose girl
who sits at the farthest end of the room.
Worry can't think.
Worry can't talk.
Worry can't do anything.
Worry sits there wondering who Worry is.

One day Worry gets sick
but the doctors don't know that.
Nobody can make Worry well.
Only Worry can.

Back home
Worry crawls out of the box she was in.
Worry breathes. Worry lives.
Worry was never meant to worry.

A well person must continue with their work schedule and
so she returns to the classroom. She can't sleep at night. The
pain in her body is unbearable. No energy, she forces herself to
school. She loves the children and wears a smile that costs her
plenty. She doesn't know she's depressed. The doctors don't
know it either. She's silent when it comes to pain, burying it all
in her body, because she once was told to live with pain. The
depression goes on for a year and a half before it lifts. She
hates not being able to sleep and so one night she gets up and
says, "I wonder if I could write. It might make the time go
quicker." She prays to God for a gift and she's amazed how
quickly it comes. The poetry flows, rivers of it. She's in touch
with the soul of herself, alive at the centre of her being. In spite
of the dead feeling in her body, she knows who she is, a woman
in touch with Divinity. For someone without a voice, you can't
keep her quiet. Her heart speaks and she listens. She knows
Truth and will record it as it's given. She's like a child with a
new toy, only this time she knows from whence it comes. No
teacher had ever imparted this kind of knowledge to her. It was
Wisdom beyond human wisdom and she would go in search of
it for the rest of her days. Nothing would cause her to deviate.
She felt whole and complete and, yet, she knew there was more
to the plan. You can't live on Spirit alone.

Unbeknown to her, she had a body that would fail her time
and again. The lessons to be learned would be anguishing ones
and there would be nothing of ego in it. Scripture fascinated
her and she wanted to live by it, taste it, feel it, know it. She
didn't realize what she was asking for when she would pray,

"Dear God, unless the grain of wheat die it shall not flourish. Please let me die in this way." She wanted to die so that God could live more fully through her. She wasn't thinking of physical death but every time depression hit her, it was like that – physical death.

Age twenty-seven to thirty-eight, she was visited by cyclic depressions. Two months out of every year she would experience this journey through hell and back, a journey she never quite got used to. Sleepless nights and days with no energy, she would turn into a zombie. Throughout her teaching years, it took incredible effort to hide her vulnerability but hide it she did. Nobody knew about the explosion of pain in her head or the anguish she was carrying in her body. It was too immense to speak of. She could have lain in bed like a bear in hibernation, but she was never one to choose the easy route. Perhaps it was pride that kept her going or the mind over matter theory she was so good at exercising.

One day she mustered up enough courage to tell her doctor what was going on. He was compassionate and told her she was depressed and that he could give her something that would help. She liked this doctor and trusted him. The medication never did work but for once she had found a doctor who could listen. A year later she came to him with the same problem. This time it was late in the afternoon. He seemed busy and frazzled. She was ready to receive help because she knew he could listen. She shared briefly but didn't feel listened to in the same way. Momentarily, he left the small office she was in and brought back a sheet of paper with questions on both sides. "Here," he said, with a smug smile, "this will fix you." And in a way it did fix her. She became silent wincing at the indignity of it all. She went away with the label, "depressed person", and chose not to go on medication because of the abnormal effects she had felt previously. She was ashamed and felt guilty about her problem. Christians are joyful people, she thought, and depression is anything but joyful. She kept the mask going for some time because she didn't want to identify with anything sad, anything opposed to her belief system. One day she would understand depression and it would turn out to be the great gift of her unfolding destiny. She would be healed and would help others on the journey but for now she still had lessons to learn.

Age thirty-eight, she arrives at the crossroads place, where she follows her heart to the breaking, despite strong opposition. Completing her seven year term as principal in Kamloops, she's going on a year of hermitage to Ottawa to pray and discern whether the Spirit is leading her away from an active religious order into a more contemplative way of life. It's one of the most difficult years of her life and the least understood. What she embarks on is the beginning of her deep healing journey, the shadowland that faces souls destined to know themselves more fully. God has a plan and it's going to be wondrous, but first she has to travel through the dark thickets of night. She's the blind daughter being led by a glimmer of Light and sometimes even that gets diminished. She would die a thousand deaths before the revelation would come but when it did come it would be worth the waiting, so glorious would be the resurrection.

The year of hermitage is horrendous, a psychological nightmare. All she wants to do is push back that which is hazardous, the repressed negative emotions of a lifetime lurking in her unconscious mind. It's a psychotic place she needs to enter but she's not ready to face the treachery of such a journey yet. In a year's time it would return with a vengeance and she would have no choice but to follow her path.

The hermitage experience turns out to be the opposite of what she thought it would be. The luxury of silence forces her to address the void within. God is with her but there is no comfort or consolation in it. She's been running from self all her life and this time she can't avoid the woman she's meant to meet. Her lifestyle has been reduced to simplicity. She's living in the basement of a boarding house in a single unit room. There are young university students on the other floors and it is often noisy, especially at night when she wants to sleep but frequently can't. Her clothes and material possessions are few, her food menu sparse. It is often cold and uncomfortable in her room but she chooses to live this way to get a feel of how the poor do it. Each day, she spends much time in prayer. She participates in Eucharistic celebrations at St. Paul's University and elsewhere. Some people ask her what she's doing. She shares her experience and some ask to come and pray with her. She welcomes them and knows God is calling her to be present to people in need. By the end of the year, she realizes the Spirit is leading her back to her active order with a new set of values. More than material poverty, it's an inner stripping of soul she's being asked to look at. She comes away from hermitage knowing she needs more prayer and solitude in her life. Her love for God and people continues to be immense and she knows it's inextricably connected with her call to serve.

During her year of hermitage, she wants to write poetry but nothing comes. She realizes her gift is totally dependent on the Spirit and in no way can she force the hand of Divinity. The creativity she longs for is held in limbo until late spring. One day, quite unexpectedly, she's sitting at her desk when suddenly she sees the sketch of a woman on the white paper in front of her. She quickly draws it and feels her entire soul go into it. Once again the Spirit visits her and the sketches keep coming over a period of six weeks. They are astonishing visions where all the moods and emotions of the human soul are being expressed through her. Each time she lifts her pencil she feels a Hand guiding her and it is with gratitude she lets herself be led. It's a transcendent and holy experience. God is with her and she is with God. Fourteen years later she would understand the meaning behind the sketches and would begin to tell the story of this woman's healing. It would be in poetic form this time, and she would write two books, *Sojourner, Know Yourself,* and *Moving On.*

She had lived simply and poorly and had learned much in her year of hermitage. The ego had been stripped down to nothing and her desires were God centered ones. She returned to her active religious order and became the principal of a school in Victoria.

THE CRUSHED SPIRIT

She'll never forget age thirty-nine, the year of the monumental breakdown where she falls apart in front of God, country and everyone. It's a great lesson in humility. One day she's the principal of a school and three months later she's like a two year old who can't put her words together. She's undergone two serious surgeries in five months and suddenly her body collapses from under her. She comes out of the anaesthetic hyperventilating, hallucinating with weird sounds going on in her head. The doctors and everyone don't know what to make of her. She's acting bizarre. Some people try and curb her behaviour. She doesn't like it when people say nasty things to her but she swallows it like a good girl should. She can't scream but wishes she could. "These damn people," she says, "they don't understand a thing of what's going on within me," and it's true, they didn't.

Her ears are exploding, popping. One minute she hears music on the radio and the next minute she hears nothing. Everything is out of balance. People coming toward her are like giants. Something has happened to her vision. It's all distorted. She remembers how it was when she was six years old, the nightmares she had where everything was huge and she was small, only this time she was smaller. People want to help her, snap her out of what she's in, but the indignity of the way they do it causes her to regress back to an experience in the womb. She sees a vision, a terrifying one of a baby just born with its head hanging down. The baby looks dead. It's herself at birth. Perhaps this explains the pressure she's been feeling at the base of her brain stem all these years. No scientific proof, but sometimes, she's told, the use of forceps does this to a person. She feels terror in her body, immense terror, but she dismisses the experience. She looks at everybody around her who has it all together and pushes the terror back in her body. So far back it will never get out if she has her way. She hates some of the treatment she's receiving but because of her loyalty she'll never say a word to anyone.

Some of the theories of psychiatry may be good for certain people but for her they have the opposite effect. Act like a baby and we'll treat you like a baby only causes her to regress more into her shell, back to the time when she was an egg in the womb and perhaps further back than she would like to remember. It's terrifying the psychological impact of this kind of journey. She's always been a squashed person but this time there's nothing left. She's been stripped of everything. God alone suffices. She hates her passage but believes in it and waits upon it for the lessons to be learned. The spirituality of Jesus is strong within her, "Father, forgive them, they know not what they do." She enters the tomb, like Jesus did, and wishes resurrection could come in three days but for her it will take another seventeen years. Patience is all part of it.

She's sent to an internal specialist for further scrutiny. This doctor is kind, so kind she could kiss his ear off. He understands her plight and assures her it will take a long time but she will get through it. She lives off this kindness for three years and every time she thinks of this doctor it's a positive energy that makes her feel well. The doctor is a modern day Simon of Cyrene who came to her in her hour of need. After three years when her energy comes back, she writes this doctor a letter to thank him for his great gift. She only saw him once but he understood her in a way few could.

When one has a crash landing, such as she did, counselling is an important part of the journey back. When she met with her counsellor, she developed certain skills that would help her on her way. She became assertive and realized that not even the counsellor could understand the gamut of what she was going through. She would speak her truth and the counsellor would often misinterpret it. This broken woman resisted statements like, "You've been a warped person all your life." It might have been true what the counsellor was saying but she felt it could have been delivered more delicately. Her poetry was also scrutinized and held questionable. She wanted to bury this gift forever, throw it away, mutilate it. To reject her poetry was to reject her. A small voice inside said, "Don't do that.

Your poetry comes from your Creator. You know the Truth. Live by it. Wait for the answers to come." The road was definitely that of the "via negativa", a passage that would one day turn into the most positive energy of her life. She needed to feel boxed and labelled in order to get in touch with her personal power. The counsellor was giving her a gift that only in retrospect would she recognize. For her, it was always a matter of integrity that she listen to her heart but even more so now when she was scraping the bottom of the bucket to restore her self esteem. Somehow the counsellor reminded her of her mother, an authority figure she needed to break loose from. She loved her mother but she had come to the point where she wanted to be her own person, distinct from everyone. In her short lifetime, she had too many people telling her what was wrong or needed fixing. She had come to the end of her tether and just wanted to be accepted for who she was.

Whenever she became assertive, she felt like a small child learning to talk for the first time. Her voice was shaky but it was her voice and not her mother's. When she visited her doctor it was the same thing. Her voice was barely audible. Her doctor was definitely compassionate but sometimes he would say things that made her cringe and, so, she was afraid to say how she really felt. Medication wasn't helping at all and, so, she explored reflexology to see if it would bring her some relief, which it did. She mentioned this to her doctor and he laughed arrogantly in her face as if she had been to some kind of a quack. She felt smaller than small and more stupid than stupid. There was a terrible dilemma going on within her. Back specialists at age fifteen had told her to live with her pain and this doctor said "scoliosis doesn't cause you pain." Because of the vulnerability of her breakdown, she felt she was imagining the pain and that it didn't exist in her body at all but why, then, was her body killing her?

She felt terribly alone and once again lost her voice to this doctor who seemed so cold and distant when she complained of anything physical. From then on, she met with him once a month and said she was doing fine. She preferred to play the game of denial and endurance rather than be ridiculed for saying how she felt, especially if the judgement was it's all in your mind. Truly, she felt like an insignificant number in a scientific medical world that was bleeding her heart to death.

Part of her therapy was to get back to work as soon as she could. She hadn't been working for five months and it was time for her to appear back on the scene. Her mind wasn't functioning well and her body registered pain all over. She didn't know how to say, "I'm not ready. I don't have one ounce of energy left," and, so, she returned to the school where she had been principal the year prior. She took on the position of school secretary for the remainder of the year and taught religion to a grade three class. It was the most gruelling experience of her life.

One day, the principal asked her to compose a letter she wanted to send home to the parents. It was a relatively simple letter but one she was unable to construct. She could no longer put words together in a sentence. She was terrified and humiliated when she exposed her difficulty. Had she been in another situation, she would most probably have been fired on the spot but this principal was kind and understanding. Teaching religion to the grade three class was equally frightening. The children knew more than she did and her facility with the English language was nil. Every time she spoke, she felt like a three year old with sawdust in her mouth, delivering a message that was empty and void of meaning. In her desperation, she prayed to God that somehow these children wouldn't be damaged by her stupidity and that the Spirit would touch their hearts in spite of her inadequacy. I guess this must have happened because the children were affectionately telling her they loved her. Perhaps God was sending these wee folk to help mend her anguish.

Her relationship with the teachers and parents was poignant. Some understood her, others didn't. It was a trying time that cost her, her life's blood. She kept on going because there was nothing else she could do. She had always been looked on as a sunshine person but this time the umbrella was up and the masks were down. She was too drained to keep on pretending nothing had happened. Her spirituality was changing, too. She was a hunk of clay allowing the Potter to shape and fire her in ways not of her own making. Where it would all lead, she had no way of knowing. She only knew she was being led by Someone greater than herself.

In the autumn of that year, she began teaching a grade one class. In spite of her minimal energy, she loved the children and gave them the best of everything she had to give. It was a difficult year but the parents and children were so affirming and gave her the motivation to continue on her mysterious journey.

She still knew that things were far from healthy in her body even though she had been congratulated by her religious community for recovering so rapidly. Daily, she was becoming more assertive and liked the new self that was emerging. She was learning to live within her limitations and was no longer aiming to please anyone. She knew how to set boundaries and began to listen to her body in a new way. There was a strong, positive self image growing in her. She even liked being small. It didn't matter what people thought about her anymore because she was satisfied with being herself. She felt her doctor was more compassionate, too. In fact, everyone was more compassionate because she was more compassionate.

During this time, she still carried an explosive energy in her body. The level of pain was high and, at times, it felt like her head was ready to blow off. In 1990, she addressed the severity of her pain in a poem called "Wind Daughter".

WIND DAUGHTER

She stood there, a small shred of a thing
as the wind tore into her without mercy.
"Oh Mother Wind," she cried,
"in the heart of a sobbing tree
you bring rain upon me."
"I do that," she said,

"for without this burden
how else can the torn face
of a rag doll get ripped?"

"But Mother Wind," I cried,
"I want to be real! Make me real!"
"Suffering will make you real," she said.
"Just listen to the harsh voice
of a howling wind
and know you can't always
stop the hand that hits you, not always."

"I love you, Mother Wind," I said,
"but you tug hard
at the roots of my knotted hair
and like the slit of a cold knife
going into me
it hurts where you enter."
"Yes, my child," she said.
It hurts where I enter.
Pain always hurts."

Grief knew no words
and I was silent before her.
"Wind daughter," she said, "you are real.
This last ache has made you real.
Go now to the others."

One day the pain would leave her body but first she would
have to go through an excruciating passage of release which
would prepare her for the knowledgeable and compassionate
healer she would become. When she spoke of her condition to
the doctor, he had a brain scan taken. Nothing showed. The diagnosis remained the same, "depressed person". She didn't like
the label and if she wasn't in a slump it was enough to put her
in one. This time the diagnosis was inaccurate and when she
returned to his office complaining that she could not move her
neck, he named it "wryneck". She liked this diagnosis better
than the first one. Living inside her body continued to be a ter-

rible struggle.

The tension mounted and by age forty-seven, she revealed her desperation once again. She really liked her doctor and trusted him even though he kept diagnosing the same thing. Finally, the doctor said she had a biochemical imbalance and that most probably she should be on medication for the rest of her life. She was excited with this new diagnosis. Biochemical imbalance sounded better than depression and, so, she went on the drug prozac for a year and a half. Waiting for the great miracle, she was disappointed to find out she felt no different from the day she went on this drug until the day she came off. Hers was a mysterious passage the medical world could not tap into.

Age forty-nine, she found herself embarking on another journey. The traditional road of western medicine was not answering her needs. She had always been intrigued by Jesus' message, "Physician, heal yourself," but had never come close enough to let it touch her. She knew Jesus was a radical man but to make a bold statement like this, she thought, could put a big portion of the medical world out of business if what Jesus said were true. It might not make the doctors happy, either, if a large number of people started pioneering their own healing. For her, there was no other option. Her pain was escalating and she needed relief.

THE SURRENDERED SOUL

The first answer came on an eight day retreat where she heard the words, "Surrender your body to me." She couldn't say whether it was God's voice speaking directly or her own. It didn't matter because the truth that was in this statement was enough to turn her entire life around. For eight days, she sunk deep into her body, so deep that she hit the rock bottom place where Divinity dwells. It was a searing experience like the incision of a knife going into her. For the first time, her body spoke and she listened. "Dear friend," it said, "you have abandoned me for so long. Listen to me because if you don't, you'll die before your time is up." She could feel every cell in her body straining to live. "Dear body," she said, "what you have been carrying is enormous, enough to flatten you, but I beg you, teach me, heal me, walk with me from this day forward." It was as if a marriage had taken place. She was in love with her body and her body was in love with her. The Divinity and she were one. She could feel the tension leaving her body, a small trickle of it, sufficient to let her know the path that lay before her. The recurring depressions she had been so frequently visited with would no longer be a pattern of her life. It was a June day and it would continue to be that from now on. She expresses her new found knowledge this way:

JUNE DAY

In my kitchen
I stopped despairing
the day when the dead song
of a whipped bird left me.

It was a June day
when the wasps
flew in at the window
and not one of them
stung me,

32

a June day
when the weakened bird
got lifted
and the rose
stuck out its stem
for the first time.

A day like today
where I rejoice and give thanks
that in my kitchen
hope rises like steam
as I burst through yet another year.

Her body did not tell her how long and arduous it would be. It just said, "Come with me. I am the way, the truth, and the life." To apply Jesus' words to her bodily experience may sound heretical but she can assure you there is nothing heretical in it. The unconditional Love energy that was in Jesus is in all of us. It's God's energy, and to be in harmony with this energy, to surrender to it, is to be restored to a sense of wholeness and well being, which leads her into telling you about the cellular story her body would have to pass through.

Her first cellular lesson began when she returned to teaching a class of grade one students after her retreat was over. She was already in the surrender mode, already into deep healing and she didn't want to put the lid on all this repressed stuff that was coming. The reality was twenty-five children were tugging at her apron strings and they needed her attention, now, not tomorrow or the next day, but now. How would she cope with this new situation when her pressure buttons were being pushed to the limit? Could she be happy and go with the flow? Would she stand her ground and know that she was just as dedicated if she left the classroom at 3:30 pm rather than 5:30 pm? What would the principal think and her colleagues and did it really matter? Could she do away with her workaholic mentality once and for all? Could she honour herself sufficiently this time to heal? The choice was hers and the commitment timely. Each day she left the classroom early and returned home to explore the deeper meaning of the words, "Surrender your body to me." All she had to do was fling herself down on her bed, let go completely, and the process would begin. Release and refuelling were happening and she was praying in a new way. The chatter in her mind was silenced and replaced by, "Be still and know that I am God." It was contemplation in and through her body. She was being healed and she knew it.

As part of her healing, she also received treatments from a gifted shiatsu therapist who helped her immensely. The damage was deep and she was ready to address the trapped emotion that lay buried in her body. It reminded her of a poem she had written in 1963.

BRUTAL WATERS
Buried
deep within you
a shipwreck
known only
to the winds of the sea.

The shiatsu treatments were always a blessing.

Perhaps, now, is a good time to talk about her vocation as teacher. In her twenty-seven years of working with children, she often felt that these small folk entrusted to her care taught her as much as she taught them. Having tasted the negative side of a school system, she wanted every child she taught to feel loved and affirmed. She wanted school to be a happy, good place for them and she wanted their gifts to be recognized. She was amazed at the beauty and spontaneity of the children she was working with. They were natural and free, something she had never known in her childhood. It was like being in a therapy session all day long. She knew about left brain thinking but these tiny folk were having her tap into the right brain side of herself. Like them, she was becoming alive and creative. She could sing, dance, hop, jump, play. She could do anything they could do. Even on a cloudy day, they could whistle up a tune and bring merriment into the room by just being themselves. She hadn't learned how to do this in the adult world, yet, but one day she knew she would. She had never done her own inner child work but here it was being handed to her on a sparkling platter. Through these beautiful children she was returned to her roots so that her early child-hood experiences could be healed. In the following poem she describes the gift these children gave her.

CHILDHOOD REVISITED AND HEALED

I want to go back and love
the shadow of that small girl
running through
a crooked patch of the earth,
to tell her
that instead of a straight path
the road ran sideways through her.

I want her to know
that I remember the time
when it was cold out
and she didn't deserve to be there.
I loved her then,
but like a thin, shelterless tree
I was not ready
to put my arms around her.

I want to go back to that small,
loveable girl
to tell her to come in out of the rain
up out of the muddy flats
onto the dry forested land.
I want to say to her,
little ice daughter
with the rain-pierced face
of a sun girl
I never disowned you then.
I would never disown you now.
And when the last wind shatters you

I want you to come out
of this blackened sky
wearing white.
I want you to come home to yourself
you, sun daughter of an earth woman,
you, pink bud,
climbing through the green clump
of your loveliness
you, child of a woman
I have grown to love.
I want you to come home to yourself.

It all seemed so easy, now, and perhaps this was the breather
she needed before getting into the deeper plunge called sink or
swim. She loved these children and they loved her.

THE PIONEER HEALER

Age fifty, she felt a compelling new call of the Spirit urging her into a healing ministry. She had no idea what this could mean or what would be the far-reaching ramifications of it. Once again, she felt like the blind daughter being led into unknown territory and she prayed for direction. Her religious community supported her decision to leave teaching for a year to explore whatever this gift of God might be. As apprehensive as she was, she was soon led by the hand of the Almighty One into a plan that was bigger than anything she could have fathomed.

A year prior to her leaving the classroom, one of her sister friends had encouraged her to have a Reiki treatment. She told her she didn't feel this was where the Spirit was leading her. "Fine," her friend said, "but I want you to know it's been one of the most gentle and powerful healing experiences of my life." She dismissed what her friend said but was curious about her raving affirmation. When she left classroom teaching the following June, her curiosity led her to have her first treatment. She was astonished at the simplicity of this healing art and wanted to find out more about it. She read Hawayo Takata's story, the woman who brought this gift to the Americas. She was truly inspired and found herself praying to God, asking that she, too, might be the recipient of such a gift. Soon afterwards, she took her first level of Reiki and realized the Source of the gift. It was Divine energy, God's love flowing in and through us. Like Jesus, we were the vessels through which God's healing was being channelled. At all times, she felt the Christ Presence with her.

People began coming for treatments. Right from the beginning, it was clear to her it was not herself but God's energy bringing the healing. Every time she treated someone, she received confirmation about the healing that was happening and because of this she was led to pursue the gift further.

There were some people in the Christian community challenging her, saying that she had moved into something occult and satanic. The word Reiki, they said, never did appear in Scripture so what was she doing promoting something that could be evil and detrimental to people's lives. She continued to discern the purity of the gift. Not only was Reiki healing others but it was bringing her own profound healing. It was a matter of integrity that she continue with the gift. Becoming a teacher and practitioner of it, she would show how this ancient healing art, God's gift to a Buddhist people, could actually enhance what we have in our Christian tradition. She had not planned to go through an eastern door. She was led there. It reminded her of Bede Griffiths, a Benedictine monk who went to the east to find the other half of his soul. She had gone to the east to find the missing tool of her healing.

The further she went with this healing art, the greater became her desire to have God take over her life completely. After ten months of deep and wonderful healing, she was shocked to awaken one morning to a crippled body. The pain had overtaken her from the top of her skull to the base of her left foot. It was like a sharp dagger going through her every time she sat, walked, stood or lay down. She remembered how it was in her teenage years. It was the same pain her body was experiencing, only this time it was worse, much worse. What was God trying to tell her now?

In agony, she returned to the medical world. Pain killers, anti-inflammatories, she was ready to take anything to relieve her. Her doctor seemed less sympathetic this time but he did prescribe medication. Nothing worked and, so, she sought help from a physiotherapist who was appalled at the disfigurement in her spine, and the terrible misalignment that had occurred through the years. The physiotherapist truly wanted to help her and suggested she ask her doctor for an X-ray. He sarcastically laughed and with a certain amount of arrogance said, "You don't need an X-ray. It won't show a thing. Your spine is deteriorating." The physiotherapist had also done some cranial sacral therapy on her and she wanted to show her doctor the literature she had on this healing technique. He said he wasn't interested and didn't want to read about something that hadn't been scientifically approved. For the first time, she felt her rage with the medical world. It was also triggering the rage she should have felt at age fifteen but didn't. What this doctor was giving her was the greatest gift of her life. It was the wake-up call that made her more convinced than ever that her road would be one of complementary healing. She would never abandon western medicine entirely but she would find her answers outside this system. Because of this experience, she found her voice and changed doctors.

Thus began the most innovative and wondrous passage of her life, age fifty to sixty-one. She had no book to guide or lead her. Just Spirit. Just body, as faithful companion, telling her what to do.

The physiotherapist continued to work with her. She was a compassionate and informed healer. "Have you ever been through birth trauma," she said, "or any other kind of trauma?" She gave her a couple of articles to read on people whose backs had seized up. After reading the material, it became apparent to her that she had been through trauma, terrible trauma. The breakdown at age thirty-nine was trying to tell her something about the severity of her condition but she had pushed it all back into her body thinking the problem lay in her mind. Now, she was being returned to the place that never had been healed.

Would she remain at point zero, a timid explorer of her existence, or would she push her voyage over the edge? Would she become stationary, stuck in her way, or would she take courage by the hand and dive deep enough to breathe sea air into her lungs? Would she? Would she? There was no other choice this time but to go forward, to take the deep plunge as her body instinctively cried out, "I am the way, the truth and the life. Listen to me and I will lead you to the fullness of your powers. I am your friend, your soul mate, your teacher, your guide. Listen to me and I will lead you." She looked in the mirror and saw her who needed healing. From then on, it was as if the entire universe came toward her on bended knee. All the right things began happening. Persons to assist her in her healing journey were sent at the right time and the right hour. There was no question in her mind. The plan was providential and she would surrender to it.

The next time she met with her physiotherapist, it was suggested that acupuncture might reduce the severity of the pain and get the energy flowing more freely. It did just that. After eight treatments, she realized she was only beginning to tap the surface of her healing passage. The truth she was being called to look at was astonishing. She had spent a lifetime burying her grief and, now, it had come back to haunt her. Her tongue was white, coated with rage. She had heard about dogs frothing at the mouth. This time it was no dog but herself that had done it to her. There was no quick fix for a journey like hers. It took a year before the white coat lifted and this was only the first layer of a million others that needed to be uncovered. There was no respite from her journey. Night and day the surrender was on and the repressed feelings kept coming. Fear, anger, grief, shame, you name it. She had never entered a wasteland as toxic as this. Her body said, "Drink water," and she drank water, gallons of it. Still, her mouth was dry and her tongue metallic. This was cellular journeying at its best. Her history was written into every pore and fibre of her being.

In her darkest hour, she met a chiropractor who was sent to assist her. He was a true healer and his compassion wondrous. He understood the journey of regression and said she would most probably have to return to the root of where her problem lay. Crippled and bent, it was like walking around in her teenage body all over again, only this time, she held the key that would eventually lead to the unlocking and straightening of her spine. It would be, not one, but a community of healers that would bring about this straightening. Her gratitude to these people is expressed in a poem written in 1990 before the actual straightening occurred.

STRAIGHTENED TREE GONE RADIANT

When I learned to accept
the wart, the mole,
the obstruction on my face
only then could I say
this field is beautiful,
that ocean is lovely,
but truly
I could not have said it
without you, my friends,
who have made my whole self
loveable.

In my weakness
never once did you call me
a deformity in the rain.
Instead,
you said I was the drizzle
that brings new life
to the trees
and, so,
I shot up in your presence
as one who knew
what it meant to be straightened.

Like a tiger strangled in a cage, she rarely spoke about the difficulty of her journey or the high price she had to pay. Perhaps, her most startling experience was with a sixty-nine year old Ursuline sister who had come to Queenswood for a three month sabbatical. It was not her normal procedure to judge people but this sister was different, really different. Wearing clunky shoes, a holy habit and veil, she presumed this nun would be traditional. She was not planning on establishing any kind of friendship with her and, yet, there was a divine plan about to unfold. She had heard from a lay person that this nun was a healer but didn't want to become connected in any way and, so, she watched from a distance. One day, after teaching a Reiki workshop, the pain in her own body was immense and a small voice inside said, "Traditional or not, ask this woman for help." When she met with this unusual healer, one of the first things the woman did was pull out a couple of magnets from under the top part of her dress. "Eccentric" was the first thought that came to mind but, then, came a flashback of a poem written eight years before.

MAGNET WOMAN

Wise woman
intimate
in your ways of knowing
out of the deep dark woods
you came
with your honey pot
loving the blemishes out of me.

What did I care about
my poor country, then?
Maps, locations, compasses,
what were these to me
when you were my destination?

In you
I sensed danger –
seagulls with swans
brambles with lilies –
and like a magnet
I was drawn to you.

Obedience had taught me
not to tangle my skirt
never to tangle my skirt
but you said,
"Forget the rules.
Nobody lives by them anyway.
And, moreover,
when you're finished experimenting
with all the clothing there is

you can be beautiful
even in the material of a messy rag."

Inside the room, her room,
I peered in
at the burnt hands and face
of a woman I knew to be me.
I could not say
whether it was her silence
or mine –
whoever it was it invaded me
like the mystery of a black spook.

"I am one,
I am many!" she said.
"Become like me!
Fire, wind, hail!"

She asked herself, could this be the woman God had sent to help heal her? As she continued to meet with magnet woman, it became apparent that this unorthodox healer was the woman who had indeed been sent by the Almighty One. Each time they met the unconditional love of magnet woman was there. Magnet woman helped to unlock the bondage in her body and gave her regular treatments. Her skills were many including muscle testing, acupressure and reflexology.

One day an astonishing thing happened. Magnet woman suddenly said, with great urgency, "I have to go to your right toe, left ear, right knee," and so on and so on. She would first feel in her body where the pain was being held and would instantly go to the spot that needed healing. As the pain left magnet woman's body, it would leave the body of the wounded one, too. Magnet woman said she had never been given a gift like this before but obviously it was a necessary part of the healing for her whose feelings had been so deeply suppressed. As magnet woman worked with the wounded one's legs and different parts of her body, she realized her muscles were like cement walls and they didn't give way easily. Magnet woman was like the Divine Potter softening the clay. It was a harsh journey but Love was in it, total love, unconditional love.

In exchange for the treatments, magnet woman wanted to learn about the ancient healing art of Reiki so, she too, could become a teacher of it. It was a beautiful exchange where a gift given was a gift received. When magnet woman left, it was not the end, but the beginning of further healing. The cement walls were down but there were more to come.

Through the ongoing gift of Reiki, this searching woman continued on her journey. Daily, she blessed her body with God's gift and let herself experience the prayerful, loving, healing energy of this Divine force. As she passed the gift on to others, it was returned in multiple measure. Through the many Reiki healing support groups and workshops, not only did others receive a treatment but she, in turn, received her own.

For a period of time, she also experienced a wonderful kind of healing through a male massage therapist who had received the first level of Reiki through her. In exchange for his treatments, she promised to take him through all the levels of the Reiki training. He, too, was psychic with the body and knew the exact location where she was holding the pain. His method of massage was far beyond anything she had previously known. She thanked God for the healing that came through him and for the warmth of the Reiki energy that covered her like a soft blanket.

Each time a door closed another would open. This time a woman healer came through. Touching the wounded one's throat chakra, she said: "You have to write your book. Your healing won't be complete until you do." It was as if Divine timing was alerting the wounded one to pay attention to her destiny.

This experience reminded her of a recent article she had read on Hildegard von Bingen, a twelfth century mystic and healer. In this article, Hildegard was referred to as the feather of God, and it stated that her physical pain would not lift until she wrote down her visions. As reluctant as the wounded one had been to write her own story, she found herself resonating with Hildegard's experience. She wondered what this physical pain of Hildegard's was, and if the pain she herself had experienced fifteen years ago after her wisdom tooth surgery had any connection. At the time, she remembered telling the specialist that her head, teeth, face, neck, jaws were locked in pain. He just said, "The surgery was more serious than predicted. The roots went deep down into your jaw. Don't expect healing to happen immediately." The pain almost drove her insane and she wasn't getting her sleep at night.

Then came the breakdown five months later. It was a psychological mad house. Everything had to do with the mind. The body didn't count. Today, she knows differently. The body does count and she might live to be one hundred and fifty if she honours the tabernacle in which God lives, in which she lives. Perhaps, Hildegard and she are the same. When Divinity speaks, you don't put up a deaf ear, or if you do, the message could be lost forever.

For one who had lived within the framework of the "chronic pain shut your mouth" syndrome, she had to ask herself, "Did Hildegard feel compelled to convey a message as she did? And who did she think she was, that God would speak through her? Was she being vain or foolhardy to expose her story? Should she go public with an audience that may distort the very words that would come out of her mouth?" As she reflected on the new space she was in, she could feel from the unburied depths of her soul a strong energy stirring. It was not her voice but that of the Spirit saying, "If you don't deliver your truth, you will go backward to a place in history you wish you hadn't." With each new step of the journey, she became acutely aware of the unmistakable immanence of God in the events that were occurring, in the people that were coming.

Just recently she met a doctor and his wife who were led to Queenswood in a totally providential way. When this couple arrived, she could feel the force of the Divine Presence in them. Their energy was pure and what they emanated was a deep down kind of spiritual goodness. As they began to share, she realized it was not just a Reiki treatment they had come for. It was much vaster and would involve her own healing as well. After doing individual treatments with this couple, she would become the beneficiary of having her own body sacredly touched and opened by a doctor who knew the secrets of her body, the defenses and closed off parts she had been so good at hiding. In her desire to be free, she sensed the Christ presence in him and responded to his unusual treatment. It might as well have been Jesus or the Divine Physician with her because that's what it felt like. Her body was opening under his guidance. If a doctor in western medicine had said, "Your diaphragm needs opening," she would have said, "Forget it, buddy," but when this doctor said it, she knew it to be true. For days after his treatment, her body continued to experience the amazing release of blocked energy so deep and integral to her healing.

This doctor from Nevada called himself a chiropractic physician and said he had retired from his normal career spending five months of the year in Victoria and the other seven in Nevada. He and his beautiful Spirit-filled wife were now totally committed to a Divine plan by which people were being led to them for healing, a journey not unlike her own. They attributed nothing to themselves but everything to God. They shared with her how they prayed daily to God that the patients they were meant to serve would be sent to them. While praying, they would envision the light and love of God being sent from their chiropractic office to touch the persons who were meant to come. One day an amazing event occurred. A patient, who was looking for their office which was hidden from view, suddenly saw a column of light emanating from the roof. She told her husband to turn the car in the direction of the light and to this day she and her husband remain patients and friends of the doctor and his wife.

This remarkable couple bear witness to a modern day kind of healing that happens when one prays and surrenders to the

Almighty One for guidance. She felt privileged to be with them and thanked God that there would be a continued connection. They were leaving, now, for Nevada but on their return the doctor's wife would pursue the gift of Reiki with her, so as to complement her husband's Divine calling. On parting, she felt a sense of awe as the words of Gerard Manley Hopkins came to her – "The world is charged with the grandeur of God."

Another amazing event happened just recently while she was receiving a Reiki treatment at one of the support groups. As she was being treated, she saw a small baby with a straightened spine inside her adult body. The baby was surrounded by light and she knew who she was. It was her perfect self before and after her mother gave birth. This time it was not her mother but herself giving birth to herself. The woman treating her was intuitive and seemed to know exactly what to do. Near the end of the treatment she returned to the left side of her skull. This time the energy in the hands of the practitioner penetrated through her head until they arrived at the baby's skull. The psychic pain was deep, so deep that tears streamed silently down her face. The pain began to dissipate and she could feel another of the cement walls lifting.

A couple of years prior, she had spoken with her mother about the time when she had lived with her in the womb. It was a beautiful sharing and she saw another side of her mother that filled her with immense gratitude. Her mother was a courageous woman who put up with much unpleasantness to bring her precious bundle into the world. Vomiting everyday of the nine months, she told her daughter that her pregnancy had been difficult. At the time of birth, her waters broke and she was unconscious upon the baby's arrival. In those days, forceps were used, a hidden violence that may not appear to harm a child until years later. Like her mother, she, too, came into the world vomiting and it took some time before the condition could be righted. One day, she privately spoke to her dad to verify what had happened. His account was similar and he said because of her minute size, he was afraid to touch her. She was like a piece of china, he said, that could break easily and he didn't want to hurt her. She now understood what her physiotherapist referred to as birth trauma. It also explained why she never felt bonded to her parents, physically bonded that is. To complicate matters, she had been indecently touched, not by her parents, but by others less considerate. It is not important to expose the details but she would like to share one of her poems addressing the great fear she had surrounding touch, a fear she was never released from until the time of her breakdown. Touch then became a blessing for her.

LONELY STANCE

> She came into our world
> something like an orchid
> fragilely beautiful
> but exotically different
> a stranger always,
> she ached to be born
> in some new way
> where the distance of touch
> would no longer mean
> having to be destroyed
> by someone holding her.

She had heard about rebirthing a number of years prior and thought it to be a far out idea. She now knew that some of us never can heal properly unless we return to the land of our psychological birth. The body records everything at a cellular level and carries the indelible memory of all that has happened to it. Some therapists say, "Get on with your life", but for her she could not get on with it until she returned to the root of where her problem lay. It was mind, body, energy medicine she was into. She was pioneering her own road to wellness and there was a great sense of dignity in it. At all times, she felt the Presence of a Divine healer with her.

Poetry and art were her way of letting the soul's Fire out, of letting the heart dance its Dance. The concluding poem in this chapter, "Self Portrait", enhances what she calls, her journey to wholeness.

SELF PORTRAIT

Eileen
solo singer
backwoods girl
extend to us
a trail
of your long root,
show us the tree
from which you were made.

Conceal not
the branch
of your hanging,
the rope
whose shreds
you live by.

Be for us
a sign of delivery,
a Stream
running through
the city of our concerns.

Each of us has a history to be lived, to be loved. This is hers.

MY HEALING PASSAGE

Like a dog that drags its tail, sickness followed me from the time I was very young. It was what you call emotional woundedness, a subtle kind of not well, that many in our western world suffer from. Oh, yes, we put up good fronts, happy-go-lucky people that we are, and never show our true selves to anyone.

I may be all wrong about the way us westerners live and, yet, I feel much of the sickness in our society stems from the very malady I'm addressing, emotional woundedness that gets trapped in our body from the time we're very young.

If I said to you, I don't think I'm the only golden haired daughter who looks good but is up to no good, you might call me a derogatory fool. Not a very nice name for somebody who's trying to find her way. So be it. I'm only stating a fact. There's a monkey in all of us and when we look at her in the mirror we're already on our way to breakthrough which leads me into telling you about mine.

I'm one of those female astronauts who didn't go to the moon for her answers, but I have travelled far underground to a place called resilient living. It's all about recharging one's batteries and facing one's self head on in the mirror. On first sight, I couldn't believe what I saw. A freak woman with dark eyes and a bruised smile telling me she's going to chart her own map and road to healing. I wouldn't be arguing with her this time. The blinders were down and I saw some strange kind of a Light shining out of her wrinkly, crinkly face. "Are you the Christ crucified one?" I queried. "Yes," came the answer. "I am He. You are she."

Living two thousand years after the Christ, I wondered what God had up his or her sleeve this time. "Is God an evolutionary God?" I began asking, and, if so, could the whole planet be swept up into something new? Why not, I thought. It seemed to fit with Jesus' words, "The Spirit will be sent to you and you will do even greater things."

There was no doubt in my mind, the Spirit had already done the great take over. It was like the last toot on the train. I hadn't a clue where I was going when the Conductor suddenly stepped in. I had never been good at charting my own course and to have Someone doing it for me seemed almost miraculous. I wondered about my new vocation as healer, if emotional woundedness could have been the prerequisite for it. It seems to me you fall down and limp your way into the ministry that is right for you and, so, I would say, yes, it is the plan of the great One that I walk with those who are like me.

My own journey reminded me of Simeon's prophecy to Mary, "Your own soul a sword shall pierce that the secrets of many may be laid open." I felt a kinship with this woman. I didn't like to think about the dagger in my destiny but I knew it was there.

Something else I wondered about were the quick fix healings that seemed to happen in Jesus' day. The blind see. The deaf hear. The lame walk. I, myself, would have liked a miracle like that but for me the plan was different. In the gospels, I don't remember Jesus ever speaking about holistic healing or psychological passages and, yet, I was sure this is what I was into. I loved the way the Spirit was leading me. It was like a spiritual lollipop and, yet, I must admit I was not prepared for the austerity of what lay before me.

I had already learned about surrender twelve years prior. It was like having a good long soak in the tub, listening to my body in a new way and not feeling at all guilty about being sensual. After all, God could be in the bath tub as well as in the dog house with me. I didn't have to go on drooping my tail, unless I chose to, and what good had that done me other than put me in the martyr complex of having a skinny bone when I wanted a fat one.

I wondered how people in the third world did it. I had heard about the city of joy. People with eyes shining like the sun in a world of have-nots. People in rags. People in slums. Bony people. Shrivelling people. Starving people. Dying people. At one time I had wanted to be a Mother Teresa working with the poorest of the poor in the streets of Calcutta. In the face of such poverty, everything seemed so overwhelmingly ridiculous the way us westerners do it and, yet, I liked my comfort as well as anyone. Clean clothes, swish cars, good jobs, superb food, material possessions, lavish homes, hot tubs, saunas, people bathing in the sun. You name it. We had it. Was it an upside down world I was living in or an upside down kind of a God trying to teach my deaf ears to listen differently.

I knew Mother Teresa was a pencil in God's hand and I wanted to be that too. Did it mean putting on old grubs and emptying my cupboards of the clothes that were in them? Going hungry for a day, a month, a year? Throwing out the excess furniture? What did it mean?

Returning to my original idea of surrender, I can't be certain what brought me here. Perhaps, it had something to do with being on a roller coaster most of my life, crashing into this thing, that thing and the other thing. I was into something new, now, not the Mother Teresa kind of something new, but it was new. Surrendering to the Spirit through one's body hadn't really found its way into our dictionary nor was it a part of the vocabulary of our day and, yet, I was convinced if one truly learned this art it could bring a type of healing to the planet that would restore dignity to the human person, so much dignity that we would walk around upright with the unmistakable joy of the Creator in us.

Every time I surrendered, it was like going to school all over again. Only this time there was nothing punitive in it. No teacher to slap your hands if you did it the wrong way, just Spirit undoing all the bad things that got you tangled in the first place. You didn't need high marks or a degree to enter this sanctuary. Just your body presenting itself at the door as one in need of healing. The lessons were relatively simple but difficult to endure. It was like entering a new kind of health system, putting your brain on hold and telling your head to go lay down on a pillow. It was the body's hour and the body's way of leading one into something cellular. For myself, I had no idea what I was being whirled into. Somebody once said I had the soul of an angel but this journey was anything but angelic. It went far deeper than surface bathing. It was a mouth, an estuary leading one into the polluted rivers that lie just under the body's edge.

It took me back to my early twenties when hard times were plenty. I was a young woman, then, twenty-three or so, homeless but living in a community. I was looking for something my religious family could not give me. My blood family hadn't been able to give it to me, either. I was an estranged woodpecker, going tappety, tap, tap, tap, drilling holes into trees, making rackety noises and disturbing no one but myself. Eventually, I found my kin, people like me, hungry for love and scratching up a storm when there wasn't one. It was a modern day Calcutta I was led into.

I was doing volunteer work at the Eric Martin Institute, a mental rehabilitation centre in the city of Victoria. I visited patients, some of them my age, others older. There was so much sadness here. Dirt, rubble, earthquakes, tremors in the land. What had these people been through? War, famine, plagues, I had no idea what their anguish was. I just wanted to lift their ravaged faces to the sun, but I was an outsider looking in. I had not gone far enough to comprehend the holocaust but one day I would be there with them. Shell shocked as they were, I would pick myself up out of the rubble and say, "No fire shall consume me for I already have been consumed." It was an inner warfare that would lead me to the height of my potential but for now I did not know that.

The nurses and psychiatrists seemed like deeply caring people but it seemed almost impossible to pull patients out of what they were in. I wondered about drug therapy and electric shock treatments. Could there be another way? And what about the body? Did it get healed? And the mind, what did you do with that if the soul was crying out? I liked being with these people. No mask wearing here. Just stark honesty, saying, "I am who I am." I was a compassionate presence to them but certainly had no solution as to what would make them well.

I remember one woman in particular, a beautiful twenty-two year old girl, thin and flat-chested, with the look of a forlorn child in her. It could have been myself at twenty. One day she had a free pass and invited me to her home. The mother was distant and the daughter turned into a raging stallion. The more she screamed at her mother the greater the distance grew. There was nothing here but a volcano between them. Better than a deep freeze, I thought, but how do you solve this kind of woundedness? It felt like I was on the hot seat and all I wanted to do was vacate the place, go out the nearest exit. I had read about mother daughter issues and knew I had my own to resolve. Perhaps, what this young woman taught me was, "Violence breeds violence. Don't blame your parents but love yourself enough to get it together." Easier said than done, I thought, but I did remember the wisdom when my turn came.

This young woman was holding up a mirror for all of us saying, parental rejection, or any kind of rejection is enough to destroy us. What she hadn't come to terms with was the gift on the other side of the fence. Whether she found it, I'll never know because my hour and time had come to do my own exploring.

After five years of walking with these amazing people, I left the city of my birth to go on my own journey, a journey that would eventually lead to the gift on the other side of my fence. St. Augustine referred to it as, "The heart is restless till it rests in God." It took two breakdowns and thirty years of zigzagging around the continent before I got to any sensible destination.

On route, and in my travels, I met many men, women and children who were not unlike the woman I had met at Eric Martin. Thirty years later, in a poem called "Sugarless Candy, No

Substitute For Love," I wrote about the poignancy of their experiences, the poignancy of mine. The poem is not a death wish but a wake-up call.

SUGARLESS CANDY,
NO SUBSTITUTE FOR LOVE

Pushed down,
fallen,
under the weight of a mountain,
sometimes Canadian girls
born into Canadian families
don't make it.

Their mothers say,
"Now dear,
you have everything
a third world child doesn't
food, clothes,
toys, games, money,
bracelets, earrings, necklaces –
everything a third world child doesn't!"

"Yes, mommy," they say,
"cock-a-doodle-doo!"
and go to bed hungry
as a chewed up rooster.
You can't fool these girls!
They know
when a chocolate
turning over in its sleep
isn't real.
Insipid
as day old phlegm
in the throat,
there is no substitute
for love
when it goes down
like a sugarless candy!

Were you to ask these girls
"What is a heart?"
they would cry,
"A bell clanging
homesick
for its mother!"

    I wondered if this poem was addressing what Mother Teresa spoke about as our Calcutta in the Americas, a subtle kind of poverty that is hidden under the wealth of our nation. I'd like to venture, she's right, but how do you heal the unhealable? Is there some kind of homework we all have to do?

    For the last ten years, I've been doing mine, roaming around in a place called purgatory, one step higher than hell. It's a wonderful space to be in and I'm getting to be an old crone at it. Thanks to my body, the teacher, the temple, the sage, I've been led into the most amazing journey of my life. History gets recorded in a variety of ways. Usually the head, the smart one, picks up a pen and writes it down. Can you imagine a body articulating the same thing, only doing a much better job of it and getting A plus, plus on the exam?

    That's the way it is when you get into cellular history. The body is a store house of incredible knowledge but if it's a wounded store house you can end up on death row sooner than you think. From the time I was a small child, my body had been on overload collecting too much trauma, too much negative, too much of those repressed feelings and hurtful memories. Too much. Too much. Perhaps, the only way my body could save me, was in the collapsing spurts it would do. Being a slow learner, it took having a crippled spine before I could begin the journey of 'uncripple'. I've hinted at the passage before, "Surrender your body to me." God only knows, I didn't bank on an eleven-year plan, twenty-four hours a day, seven days a week, three hundred sixty-five days a year, without respite even on a Sunday.

    Releasing all these repressed feelings was like going

through a manure pile to find the orchid. I don't know why I had to go through these muddied waters to get the exquisite best out of everything. It's like the dull pearl and the exotic go together. I think it has something to do with the inevitable death-resurrection cycle Jesus spoke about. You pay the price and get the goods.

I'd like to share a little more about surrender because I think it's the key issue in saving us from some of the common diseases of our day. Arthritis, fibromyalgia, chronic fatigue syndrome, depression, Alzheimer, strokes, cancer; the list is endless and it doesn't seem to be a matter of age when the body turns sour. As I look out at a broken world, I feel at one with the travailing universe. There's an empathy in me, because like them, I'm one of the wounded ones who's climbed into her coffin often enough to know the downward drag, the body's tomb hole that can't do anything but scream the death scream. Why I'm being blessed at this time and this hour, I'm not quite sure. I only know I'm one of the fortunate ones on the up side of things and I'd do anything to get everyone out of the doldrums, if I could. Of course, the "Mrs. Fix It" syndrome doesn't work on anybody but one's self and, perhaps, this is the best clue I can give.

Back then, to the idea of surrender. How do you get there if you're in a full time ministry? Do you shut the door and say, "Sorry folks, I'm going home to bed," or do you face yourself honestly and put up with the unpleasantness that goes along with this kind of journey. I'm not talking about surrender, as in war, where the other side wins but, rather, an inner warfare where the victor is you and only you. All of us are made of energy, Divine energy, but when the system gets blocked we could be chugging along at zero and end up in a place called stink hole. No mileage left, no one to rescue us. From my own experience, it's the best place one could be. Yes, blessed be that stink hole that sets us free.

There's a tragic lover in all of us and it's up to us to find her, which brings me into the active, passive quality of surrender.

It's akin to a woman with a hot iron. She feels the scald under the skin, dips down into the passive zone called repressed feeling, and lets it come, one blast after another. Not a mini blast but a ten year one.

We sometimes talk about toxicity in the air and in the food we eat and, I suppose, sickness does have something to do with the foul atmosphere and the not so good nutrients coming into us. But let's take it one step further. Suppose we look at the toxicity of buried emotion. It could be the dynamite stick we're most afraid of, the calamity of calamities. As much as I hate to admit it, the dynamite and I are one, which brings me to the point called active recovery. The best image I can think of is Mrs. Porcupine, prickly all over, and having her quills pulled out. Active recovery is like this. It has nothing to do with soft, cuddly bears or sucking the sweet juice out of your thumb. That's why Reiki, the healing ministry I've been led into, is such a blessing. It prepares you for the worst and the best. On the one hand, it puts you on cloud ninety-nine with your Maker, a positively delightful experience of Divine energy flowing into you - the luxury of passive surrender. But get ready. There's a hook on the line. It's the active side of Reiki which says for every angel there's a demon. You may say, "Oh, no, I'm too pure for that," or "give me the easy way out," but if you're anything like me, you'll shut up and do your homework.

Spit, rant, rave. Swim it out. Walk it out. You'll do whatever you have to. It's your body that wants and needs the healing. Taste your anger. Feel your anger. Know your anger. Push your anger out. There's no room for discouragement here. Just hope. Plenty of it. After the thorn comes the lily. So get on with your passage. It's the love, hate, love walk that only you can do.

Surrender takes you out of the driver's seat into a whole new way of being. Heart, body, mind and soul, they all get in on the jig. It's the Divine plan where everything starts coming toward you. All life is a flow. You don't arrange too much of anything. You just get led. People arrive at your doorstep and you know what to do. Events occur and you go with them. Being this kind of a vessel, I guess I'm in a kind of privileged position. On the receiver's end, I'm getting all the healing I need, and on the giver's end, I'm no more than the channel through which God's healing flows.

It's complementary healing and preventative medicine I'm into and this time I know I'm nobody's dumb bunny. I'm kissing my own body well. No doctor could do it for me. Just me, myself and I, and, of course, the great One, the mighty Physician of us all. My spine is straightening and I know it. My chiropractor knows it, too. The ugly duckling is turning into a beautiful swan. I look different, feel different, am different. My energy is positive. My attitudes, values, everything about me is changing. I've lived long enough in the bucket of stress to know not to go there ever again. The "How To Books" tell us it's one of the biggest killers of our day, so why put ourselves at this kind of risk?

Getting back to the whole notion of disease, there's so much to look at. Sometimes it doesn't make sense why you're sick and I'm well. Why this person has cancer and that one doesn't. And, then, there's the whole mortality issue. Why does the baby in the crib die suddenly and the grandpa in the rocker live on to one hundred? There are so many unanswerables and to blame God for any one of them is to miss the whole point of the great Light at the end of the tunnel.

I've heard it said that anger is at the root of most diseases and if we can catch it soon enough, siphon it off, get it out of our system, then perhaps we'll be a healthier people. I know this to be true for myself, Miss Pussy Cat going around with her soft feet, licking up the cool water, when what she wants to do is hiss off the steam. I'm getting good at doing my release work and at the same time feeling proud about forgiving myself and others. I don't want to put a guilt trip on anyone or make a judgement that stored anger is at the root of most illness. I'm just saying it could be. Anything toxic in our system could effect the well being of how we live. Harmful relationships, lack of meaning, high stress, unhealed emotions, low self esteem, crippling choices, negative thinking, poor diet, lack of exercise, not enough rest, little time to contemplate – all these and more could be pumping a type of poison into our blood stream that will one day turn against us. Perhaps, if we begin the reversal soon enough we'll not need plastic surgery or the kind of face lift that smacks of anything mechanical. Perhaps, we'll all turn back to the Light, to positive Energy, to healing ourselves and others, to healing planet earth and, then, move into the new millennium with renewed hope and optimism to discover a kind of wholeness we can't be silent about.

As much as we want to be well, sometimes sickness is what we're visited with. It could be a person's destiny to be stricken that way to teach us all a lesson. I once knew a man like this. He was a dear friend of mine who was visited with MS at age twenty-two. Eighteen years later, crippled and confined to a wheel chair, he delivered a message that we all need to hear. He accepted his lot in life, and his face was lit with transparent joy. His love for God was immense and his passion for life amazing. He was a man that inspired people wherever he went. The light of God was in him and he was spiritually and emotionally whole, not cured, but whole. There are so many men, women and children like him, so many Rick Hansen's out there, that we can never judge why things are the way they are. Only accept that at the heart of life there is mystery.

My own path to healing has been long and devious and perhaps, only now, am I hearing for the first time what my body has always wanted to tell me. "Dear friend," she says, "your body is like a fine tuned musical instrument. Play her well and she'll sing the melody best suited to you. Nothing is discordant to her. Your history is your history and whatever happens to you, she's the wise one, the juggler, putting it all together. Learn from her the rhythm that is best for you." I can say, "Yes, dear body, you know me. I am a small bird on a pinnacle. It is you who have helped me see the bigger picture and I am grateful to you for my handicap, the thorn under my flesh, that has led me into the most wondrous healing ministry of my life."

60

REIKI: A SPIRITUAL DOORWAY TO
NATURAL HEALING AND CREATIVITY

You might think a furnace can warm you, but when it's soul Fire, you'll know the difference. Such has been my journey as poet and Reiki healer these past ten years. Moving into an eastern healing art in a Christian setting, I have compared my journey to that of a wise baker who makes a cake the same way for fifty years. Suddenly the recipe changes, ingredients shift, and the once bland taste gets more delectable. Such has been my experience with Reiki.

As a practitioner and Christian teacher of this ancient Buddhist healing art, I have seen people's lives renewed, turned around, made whole. Simultaneously, my own radical conversion has flung me to the furthest limits of my creativity and given me new eyes with which to see. One might compare the experience to a kaleidoscope where the brilliant face of the Almighty One is reflected in every human soul there ever was or is. Through these new lenses, Divine Plan has stretched and readied me for a spiritual journey into a deeper level of consciousness. Rooted in my Christian tradition, I remain open to the teaching of other cultures that continue to inspire and enhance my own.

In the case of Reiki, when the whole of a person begins to heal, as has happened with me, there is a side of the soul that wants to do nothing else but sit before the hearth fire at night and recognize the journey for what it is. Kindled by the warmth of this Flame, my poetry and art reflect the passage of a warrior woman who has gone into battle with her lower self so that the higher God-self may emerge.

Similar to the Christian laying on of hands, Reiki is like a prayer over the entire body bringing peace, harmony and well-being. In my daily practice of Reiki, the recipient is invited to surrender to the living God within one's energy system, thereby activating the body's natural ability to heal. It is not the practitioner's energy but God's that does the healing.

61

Being connected with Divine energy in this way and open to its influence, my poems are often prophetic, pointing out the way of my journey ahead of time. The most recent powerful experience of this was in relation to my father's death. Two years prior to his going, I had written a poem entitled "Even In Death Dad's Love Will Heal." The stark reality of this event occurred when my father came out of a coma through a Reiki treatment to show us that when we meet God, the beatific vision of it can be reflected all over the human face. The radiance we saw was only one of the many parting gifts dad gave us. Here is the poem dedicated to my father, my friend, the one I loved in life and, now, in death.

EVEN IN DEATH DAD'S LOVE WILL HEAL

Black,
colour of a torn up tulip,
stick it on your father's face
until the eyes become indelible
as yours.

Genealogy has it
the daughter inherits
the look of her father.
One glance from these navy eyes
and she has the uncanny ability
to light up the dark corners
of a dim room.

They are so much alike,
father and daughter.
A small girl
somersaulting down a hill
she exudes humour
as freely as he does
only sometimes
she catches him playing
with dust balls in the thermos
as if there was something wrong
with growing old

something irreversible
as bad breath.

She can't stop loving this man
he's the only dad she has
and she'd do anything to keep him forever
relinquish calendars
turn clocks backward
put him in her pocket
with a warm blanket marked
eternal daddy.

She remembers him as he was
huge heart size of an ocean
forty years a school principal
loved, honoured, respected,
friend of children, parents
this beautiful man
falling off a pedestal
into a pit called no more.
and she wants to save him.

Daddy's girl,
mischievous monkey,
they could be twins
in the same buggy
identical shoe laces
each going their separate way
he on one continent
she on another.

Long after he's gone
she'll remember her tiny hand in his
the big finger over the little one
tracing the word love
down the side of her cheek.

By connecting with my father through this Reiki treatment, I experienced the tangibility of God's presence, and understood more fully the meaning of this Japanese word. Translated as "God conscious Energy" I realized that Reiki had become the poetry of my soul. What I write and draw is what I live. Reiki is about the whole of creation singing its song in and through us. It is about the wonder of God and the great Spirit animating every living thing.

Becoming a pioneer of my own healing, I am aware that today, more than ever, people are searching for balance in their lives, looking for doorways that will open and lead them to it. To counteract a culture of growing violence, people are looking for a new way of returning to inner peace. Having found a doorway that works for me, people often want to pursue the pathway I continue to explore.

Periodically, the phone rings and the person on the other end says, "My friend just took a Reiki workshop from you and is amazed that this healing gift of God can be passed on in a week-end in such a simple and wonderful way. Can you tell me more about it? I've been searching for something spiritual and holistic and I think maybe this is a path I want to pursue." Sometimes the voice on the other end says, "I just received a treatment from someone who took your Reiki workshop. I've never experienced anything quite like it. My body felt so blessed and renewed. I've been looking for something that could bring greater balance and wholeness into my life. Do you think Reiki might be the answer?"

My response usually is, "Yes, I think Reiki could be one way of bringing you the harmony you're looking for." In talking with people, though, I tend to avoid the simplistic answer and look at the broader picture of healing which is what Reiki addresses.

Let's look, now, at a commonly asked question, "What is Reiki and can you tell me more about it?" Reiki is an ancient Tibetan form of natural healing that assists body, mind and spirit in attaining its own highest level of healing and wellness. This healing art was rediscovered in the Japanese culture by Dr. Mikao Usui in the late nineteenth century. It is a spiritual healing gift which was passed on to Dr. Usui in a moment of enlightenment after a twenty-one day retreat on Mt. Kurama. Usui Sensei had gone there to seek direction for his life, to fast and to pray. At the end of the experience, the healing gift that was given was what he called Reiki, a Japanese word meaning, "Universal Life Force Energy." He went on to open a clinic in Tokyo in 1922 and in his lifetime passed the gift on to over two thousand people. He was loved and revered by the people of Japan and often travelled to distant towns and villages where he would teach and share this healing art which has now become a universal gift for the whole of our planet. He was a man of great spirit and is remembered for his incredible compassion which was displayed in such a beautiful way in 1922 at the time of the Kanto earthquake in Tokyo. He took the gift of Reiki to this devastated city and used its healing powers on the surviving victims. Dr. Usui died of a fatal stroke in 1926 at the age of sixty-two. Since his death, the gift has continued to flourish.

In the west, Hawayo Takata is the one who brought this healing art to us. Her own story of healing through Reiki is a miraculous one and, I believe, when God has a mission for a person, as in the case of Hawayo, something profound happens in order for the message to be passed on in a compelling way. Hawayo began her training as a Reiki healer in Japan with Dr. Hayashi in the spring of 1936 and in the summer of 1938 was initiated as a Reiki Master in Hawaii. She died in 1980 at the age of eighty and as a result of her dedication, the gift has spread far and wide through the Americas and, is now, an international blessing for the peoples of the earth.

There is a flexibility in the Usui system which makes it broad enough to include a wide range of methods and techniques while at the same time keeping the purity of the gift intact. Coming from a Christian heritage, I find that this eastern healing art enhances what we already have in our tradition. Christ touched and healed and, so, we in our day continue to lay hands on one another and pray for healing as Jesus did. A closer look at Reiki shows that we are doing the same thing, only taking it one step further. In a Reiki treatment the entire body system is treated in a holistic way and the one receiving the gift is invited to surrender to the Divine energy of God which in turn activates the natural healing powers innate in all of us. The practitioner is merely a vessel through which God's healing flows. Since no personal energy is expended, both client and practitioner receive healing from the same Divine Source and come away from the experience feeling energized and fulfilled. There is often a sense of oneness with the Creator coupled with a deep spiritual joy and calm. One woman suffering from a severe sport's injury said, "I've never felt anything so ecstatic." She went on to take a workshop in order to help others suffering from sport injuries.

As a practitioner, I always remain centred in the Christ healing energy, silently praying for the good of the person, and am aware at all times that whatever healing takes place is God's and not mine. A treatment usually lasts about one hour. The recipient remains fully clothed and lies down in a comfortable position unless for some reason sitting up is easier. The Reiki practitioner gently lays his or her hands on the body in several positions which correspond to the major organs, chakras and endocrine glands. In my own individual practice, I treat the entire body which includes arms, hands, legs, feet, since tension or buried emotion can be hidden in any of these areas. A treatment can be just as effective when given a slight distance away from the body but most people like the direct contact of hands on. Often the receiver feels heat from the practitioner's hands although sometimes it is experienced as a cool soothing energy depending on the needs of the body.

The effects of Reiki are far reaching. It can accelerate physical healing. A woman in her seventies, who broke her wrist, reported that after several Reiki treatments from her daughter, her wrist healed in three weeks rather than the expected six. She also said her wrist was totally flexible and that she didn't need therapy.

The Reiki energy is gentle and soothing but also powerful in its ability to heal. It can relieve pain and tension, and release blocked energy, bringing the body into a state of relaxation and well being. In an age of stress, it can bring peace to our bodies and harmony to our souls. It can relieve high levels of anxiety which often contribute to modern day illnesses. We can come away from a treatment feeling physically, mentally, emotionally and spiritually well. One man suffering from cerebellum degeneration described his treatment this way, "I felt like a baby in a wicker basket floating on the ocean and being looked after." Another woman describing her experience said, "It felt like warm rays going into my body and things coming out." After the treatment, she shared that she was anxiety ridden and had a sore back but, now, she felt lighter, more relaxed and pain free.

Reiki treatments are effective at any age level. Babies particularly love it. One woman shared about her niece's new born baby who was howling and agitated. The Reiki energy quieted the little one almost instantly and she became still. It was most probably as good as having a drink of mommy's milk. The niece shortly afterwards took a Reiki workshop to have the gift for herself. Another beautiful healing happened with a small six year old girl. She became frightened of her parents as they continually argued with each other and lost her voice within the family. The mother was perceptive and noticed what had happened. She brought her little daughter for a Reiki treatment and together we talked and prayed and shared. It was a sacred moment treating this small child. After it was over the little girl said, "That was nice. I felt warm and cozy all over and I'd like to come here everyday." I told her if mommy came for a workshop she would be able to do the same kind of treatments. The mother decided to take the Reiki level one training so that she and her daughter could experience healing together. The little girl went away happy and contented and found her voice once again within the family.

For those of us who practice Reiki, we remain humble and grateful before the Giver of it. The stories of quiet healings are numerous and those who come for treatments are often in wonderment at the mystery of it.

Some people come looking for a cure and what they receive instead is healing on a different level. It reminds me of a brave young man, age thirty-five, who had been struggling with a malignant brain tumour for five years. He came to see me two weeks before his death. The treatment brought him to a place of deep peace and acceptance. He felt so good after it that he thought possibly he might be cured. A year later his mother came to see me. She said, "I've come because I want to experience that deep peace my son did before he died." After the treatment she said, "I understand now."

For a year and a half, I walked with another beautiful, young woman who became a teacher for all of us. Her entire body, including her eyes, was overtaken by the insidious disease of cancer and she fought it the whole way with a hope one rarely sees. She herself, her mother, her sister, and her friend, all took Reiki in the hope she would be cured. She was not cured but Reiki brought a kind of comfort to her body that nothing else could. Everyday she experienced the gift as a blessing which made her unbearable passage more bearable. Healing also happened at an emotional level between family members. As for the caregivers, they no longer felt helpless in the face of her pain. When Reiki was administered throughout her chemotherapy treatments, she experienced no negative side effects, whereas, prior to the Reiki, she had experienced the down side of this drug. She died as courageously as she had lived, teaching us about honesty of emotion and allowing a loving community to walk with her. If anyone deserved to see the Light, she did.

Reiki, then, is not only a gift for the living but for the dying as well. Death comes to all of us and the Love that flows through the hands of a Reiki practitioner can help make the transition to our new Life easier. A number of people in the Reiki healing support groups have done volunteer work at hospice and in the cancer clinic to walk with people in this way. Within the family, it is a beautiful gift to send our loved ones on their way.

The purpose of the Reiki support groups is to continue to journey with people in a healing manner and to explore together this amazing gift of divine grace. Reiki has been instrumental in my own healing and without it my spine most probably would have never straightened or become as flexible as it is.

Animals also respond well to Reiki. It is wonderful to think Life force is in them, too, and that we can love, honour and respect them as an integral part of God's creation. One woman who took a Reiki workshop said the reason she was there was because of her pony. She owned a farm with animals and had been told by the veterinarian that her sick pony would die. A friend of this woman, who did Reiki, asked if she could treat the horse. The pony became well and, now, the woman who took my workshop, lovingly treats not only her animals but her family and friends as well. Another animal story happened with a dog that had sores all over its body. The medication that the veterinarian suggested was very expensive and, so, the owner of the dog decided to give him a Reiki treatment. The sores cleared up immediately and have never returned since. There are countless human and animal stories like this. To the skeptic it may seem, how can this be, but for those of us who have received the gift, we know the Source from which it comes. All is gift, everything is gift. We cannot make it happen, but when it does happen we are grateful.

We know that plant life benefits from Reiki, too. One of the women in our support groups did an experiment with her plants. Those that were treated flourished. The others did not. In our busy consumer-oriented world, we often get so caught up with material things that we forget the wonder of God's life-energy pulsating through the entire universe, be it in the trees, the plants, the flowers, the ocean, the stars, the planets, the animals, the humans. We are all interconnected. God is the universe at our centre and whatever Light we emanate is from the One who connects us all. The Buddhists would say we are compassionate beings and so, Reiki, the unconditional Love energy of the universe would fit perfectly into their scheme of things and into our Christian belief system, too.

Reiki is not a religion or cult nor is it in any way exclusive. It transcends belief systems and takes one to the heart of God. It cannot be contained by linear left brained information, just as the bigness and mystery of God, cannot be shrivelled into this dogma or that. It cuts through our religious interpretation of things and allows us to discover the essence and truth upon which all religions have been founded. Reiki promotes an open and creative mind and enhances our spiritual journey to know ourselves better. It puts us in touch with our inner selves, with God at our centre. From this sacred space, comes our intuitive ability to know and to heal. As we are inwardly fulfilled, our lives become a joyful expression of our Creator.

In Reiki, there is an expectation that we would improve ourselves, that we would become living witnesses of the Truth we live by. In sharing the Reiki Ideals with you, which Dr. Usui promoted as an important part of the healing system, it could be the voice of Christ speaking to us. "If this is so," people have asked me, "Why, then, isn't Christ enough for you?" In answer to them, I have replied, "It is a matter of integrity that I remain rooted in my Christian tradition but it is also a matter of integrity that I bear witness to the surprise of God who came through an eastern door to heal me while I was waiting at the western one." The Reiki Ideals, then, are just another way of calling us to fullness of being.

REIKI IDEALS

Just for today,
I will live an attitude
of gratitude.
Just for today,
I will be free of worry.
Just for today,
I will be free of anger.
Just for today,
I will live honestly.
Just for today,
I will show love and respect
for every living thing.

Reiki is meant not only for healing others but is a tool for self healing as well. Through a spiritual healing attunement, this gift is passed on through a Reiki Master teacher. Anyone, including children, can receive the gift. In fact, one of my most powerful experiences was with an eight year old girl who received the attunement and exchanged a treatment with me. The healing that flowed through her hands was overwhelming and reminded me of Jesus' words, "Unless you become like little children, you shall not enter the kingdom of God." The beauty of this healing art is in its simplicity. It goes beyond the academic mind into the realm of Spirit. By simply placing one's hands on another, the Reiki energy begins to flow and God's healing becomes apparent.

As initially stated, Reiki alone won't heal us but it certainly can be a major factor in contributing to it. Reiki is the Life force energy of God with us, a road of Light leading to balance, order and harmony but it won't happen unless we personally and responsibly participate in our healing passages. This could mean changing our lifestyles, our attitudes, our values, our goals or looking at our addictions in a new way and shedding light upon them. It may also mean additional therapy and allowing a medical world in to assist us. To be whole is to be happy and if Reiki can do that for us, then it is worth exploring this free gift of Divinity.

EPILOGUE:
HEALING IMPACT OF BODY-MIND CONNECTION

This chapter comes as an add-on, totally unexpected, but necessary to complete the journey that is mine. My book was at the publisher's ready to go when suddenly I was plunged into the most critical and dramatic part of my healing. As a result of this experience a final chapter, "Body-Mind Connection", was needed to address the unusual new direction my healing had to take.

Because of my recent discovery, I believe that what has happened in my life will begin to happen in the lives of many and that we will see the unfolding of a Divine plan that will border on the edge of spectacular. You won't find it written about in the ordinary literature of the day because it's something into which we are going to evolve. There will be some in the human family, struck down as I am, by the force of God to whom the revelation will be given. Upon entering this domain, the power of God will overtake our lives and we will become clear vessels of Divine light, love and goodness. We will be led in ways that are pure and true and the wisdom emanating from the essence of our being will be charged with joy, the joy of knowing who we are, where we came from, and where we are going.

I believe there are numerous Christ figures walking on planet earth already and that there will be more and more enlightened souls who break through old traditions to cross over into the terrain of the new. One of these healers is this Nevada doctor I spoke of in my first chapter. Little did I realize that on his return to Victoria, he would be the one to lead me into the most dangerous part of my healing journey, a passage underground where mud pies and diamonds would be found together. His name was Joshua, meaning seeker of God. I, too, was seeking God, the height and length and depth and breadth of wherever that Love would lead. For years I had been searching for the pearl of great price but never suspected Joshua would be the one to take me there. My relationship with Joshua

was like that of the woman at the well. He loved people uncon-
ditionally as Jesus did and wanted to lead them to the Eternal
Waters. He was God's gifted healer and highly skilled chiropractic physician who knew the truths of people's stories by listening to their bodily responses. Unbeknown to me, Joshua
was the one who would help me probe the depths of where God
wanted me to go. It was a body-mind journey where the mystery of God would lead us into zones where only the blind dare
tread. About a week before entering this phase with Joshua the
following poem was inspired as a signal that something was
about to happen.

BEHIND THE EYES OF THE BLIND ONE
A SUN SHONE THROUGH

The Voice came toward me.
"Blind one with the darkened eyes
let me lead you"
and I in answer said:
"even if you throw my clothes away
to be eaten by the birds
I will let you lead me!"
Sitting on the sharp edge
of a craggy cliff
I had spent my entire life-time
trying to be happy
but now it felt like the black hole
of a pit
had torn the skin away from my smile.

I could have ended my journey here
had not a strange, beautiful Hand
lifted the veil from my unseeing eyes
telling me
blindness was the cataract
I walked into.

Under the cloud
a sun came rolling in

and for the first time
I saw my Healer dressing me
in the same radiant cloth
He wore
three days after His burial.

The first remarkable incident occurred a couple of days after the poem was written. Joshua had treated me and at the end
of it had me sit down on a chair. As he looked into my eyes he
realized there was some kind of a strain and misalignment. His
diagnosis was startling: "Your glasses are harming you, Sister.
I want you to take them off and I don't want you to put them
on again until you get a new prescription. There is something
wrong in the construction of your lenses." My immediate
response was, "Joshua, if I don't wear them I'm as blind as
a bat. I can't even see you on the chesterfield and besides my
eyes were tested not long ago and everything was fine." With
a knowing smile, he insisted I follow his advice. The choice
was mine. There was nothing of arrogance in him. He spoke
from an inner authority like Jesus did. Perhaps, this was the
test I needed to trust and follow this man of God who had been
placed on my path to help me walk in the oddity of shoes most
people won't be seen tramping in. My path was different and
his was, too. In Joshua, I had a sense of the extraordinary,
somebody picked by God with a clean heart and pure soul. At
least, that's what it felt like and I chose to follow.

Without glasses, the sisters wondered why I was walking
around blind as a bat in my own home. I had already realized
that Joshua was right about the eye strain. I could feel the difference once the glasses were removed and, so, I told them my
eyes were changing and I needed to have them tested. In a
small way, I felt the handicap that blind people must feel.
However, my blindness went far deeper and unbeknown to me
Joshua would be the one to reveal it.

A week later I visited the optometrist and had my eyes
tested. The left eye definitely needed a stronger prescription
but the right lens she said was fine. I told her about the wisdom

of Joshua who said there was something wrong with the right lens in the way it had been constructed. I could tell by her disapproving glance that she was not impressed by what could be considered quackery. She checked the glasses with their machinery in the office and told me they were perfectly constructed. I wanted the new prescription for the left lens to be made immediately and, so, I went to Lens Crafters who had them constructed within the hour.

That night Joshua and his wife came to the Reiki healing support group. Feeling good about my glasses, I said to Joshua, "I have my new prescription." He looked at me and said, "Sister, the right lens has not been properly constructed. Your eye is going in the wrong direction. You need to take your glasses back and have the right lens reconstructed." "Joshua," I said, "I'm going to feel like a fool going back and telling them that I need a new lens when the machinery has already proved otherwise." He looked at me with the same knowing smile and said, "You've got to take them back."

Feeling somewhat ridiculous, I visited Lens Crafters the next day and told them what Joshua had said. They put my glasses in their machinery and the report was the same that the optometrist had, perfect glasses, perfect prescription. Because of Joshua's insistence, I told the woman I still wanted a new right lens. She said, "I won't have the lens made unless I talk with your doctor first." She spoke to Joshua on the phone who informed her that in the grinding of a lens there can be an imperfection which can cause the prescription to be slightly off centre and which, in turn, can harm the eyes.

She came back and did further testing with my eyes and indicated that, yes, she felt a new right lens was needed. Joshua said he would come down to check the glasses once they were completed. It took an extra hour for the lab to properly construct my glasses. After making the right lens, they discovered that the plastic in both lenses was too heavy and was causing some kind of an imbalance. At this point, they constructed two new lenses with lighter plastic.

Never having been to Lens Crafters before, I was impressed by the expertise of the lab technicians as well as by the clerk who assisted me. Everyone was so accommodating and they wanted to make sure I got the right prescription this time. On top of this, they did not charge me for all the extra work that was entailed. After checking the glasses and confirming they were the right ones, Joshua and I thanked them for their absolutely wonderful service.

For four years, I had been wearing the old glasses thinking they were the right ones because it was the first time I had ever worn bifocals. I thought the eye strain I was experiencing had something to do with adjusting to these new kind of lenses. With the new glasses, the strain lifted and I saw the world with greater clarity and lightness thanks to Joshua.

The next time I met with Joshua for a treatment I told him I needed to share an experience I didn't fully understand. Part of it was blissful, the other part confusing. The blissful part had happened a few days prior at a Reiki healing support group where another beautiful woman became part of a rebirthing experience with me. It was stronger and deeper than the one referred to in chapter one. As she came toward me I felt the loving force of a Divine presence surrounding my entire body. My eyes were closed and I saw standing behind me four figures of Light. She doesn't know why but as she touched my head she was led to say, "It feels like the head of a baby" and with that I was plunged into a rebirthing experience. Wherever she touched me the tears silently flowed. So loving and nurturing was the treatment that it seemed to mend every injury from the time of birth onward.

As I shared my bliss with Joshua I also revealed to him the confusion about a dramatic experience which had occurred eighteen years ago. At that time, I saw the terrifying image of a dead baby, myself hanging above my body at the time of birth. As we entered the treatment together we had no idea what was going to transpire. Joshua asked me to return to the beginning of my birth to visualize what it was like. I couldn't visualize a

76

thing and so I asked God to let me be in my body and feel what it was like from the time of conception up to and including birth. What was shockingly revealed was a new kind of awareness, that the body has a memory the mind doesn't. As Joshua took me through the rebirthing experience it became hideous, horrible and filled with terror.

Like Jesus who did bizarre things such as putting mud on people's eyes so they could see, so too was Joshua led to listen to the Spirit in an unusual way. The Voice of the Spirit within Joshua told him to pick me up like a baby. He resisted the Voice twice but on the third time felt compelled to listen. It was only at that moment when he picked me up that my body felt dead, heavy, weighted. Joshua felt the heaviness, too. He kissed me on the back of the head the way a father would a newborn. So repulsive was it that I became totally disconnected from him. There was no love, no feeling in me, just terrible resistance to a male energy that disgusted me. He put me back on the treatment table and gently covered me with a blanket. It was only at that moment that I felt a trickle of feeling come back into my body. An onlooker might say, "The both of you are stupid fools," and on a human level it would appear to have been that but on a Divine level it was the only thing that could have brought me to the healing I needed. Shocking, yes, and even more startling was the awakening that would come a few hours later. The experience left me momentarily speechless and I did not want to talk to Joshua until I had time to process it.

Joshua and his wife had invited me to a Gregorian chant concert that night at St. Andrew's Cathedral but I told them I couldn't be in the presence of people, their company or anyone's. I needed to be alone with God to digest what for me was overwhelming.

A few hours later my mind became illuminated. It was like having all the pieces of a jigsaw fall together instantly. For the first time, I saw and understood my story from birth and even before birth until now. Another prophetic poem surfaced and I was compelled to put it to paper.

A SEER LIVES INSIDE THE HIDDEN HOLLOW
OF THIS CAVE

I've travelled far to get here
but never have I seen anything so strange
as this seer in a cave
sitting still in a chair bending backwards
when she wants to go forward.
Going in opposite directions to ours
she could be a dumb pigeon
paddling her way home
or more likely
a young girl with an ancient existence
humming her song into the trees.

Guided by the Spirit of an eagle
she's a woman now
gone back to her origins
to see things we don't,
boots, bonnets, petticoats -
her body knows what it was like
before she began falling back
into the womb of her mother.

The water was pure then,
and the rain came trickling down her face.
She loved everything
the soft skin of humans, rabbits, birds, deer.
In the sweet scent of a rose
she could smell the essence of her being.
The sky was bluer in those days,
the sun brighter.
The universe was filled with light
and the Divinity was in her.

Suddenly, the breakdown at age thirty-nine made sense, total sense. I saw with clarity, now, my destiny as a healer. There were others out there undergoing similar struggles as mine and I was able to assure these people not to be afraid of their inner earthquakes. If they registered off the Richter scale, as mine did, it didn't have to mean they were going insane but rather that they were coming into a new level of maturity. The spiritual journey is like that - the deeper the roots, the taller the trees, the greener the growth. The gift Joshua gave me was to unleash the trauma that I had so cleverly pushed back into my body at age thirty-nine, the trauma of birth and so many other traumas I had been sitting on unknowingly.

In talking with Joshua about this startling experience, he shared with me that in his twenty-one years of treating people he had never been led to do anything so radical as to lovingly carry and rock me in his arms. I was grateful that he had had enough courage and love to risk following the Voice, the same Voice that had spoken to me a week prior: "Blind one, with the darkened eyes, let me lead you." Because of my implicit trust in Joshua as a healer, I had surrendered myself to the unusualness of what happened. Had it been anyone other than Joshua I would have been off the table and out of the room in a flash.

Joshua had taken me to a place where I would now need help to release the further trauma that was surfacing in my body. Once again a Christ figure came toward me in the form of a woman who knew about the excruciating journey through birth trauma because of her own. The gift she shared was that of cranial sacral therapy. I had two powerful and lengthy treatments with her. It was true my body knew how to unlock itself from its entrapment but I needed her assistance to facilitate the opening that was required before my body could do its work. It was an immense journey backwards before I could go forward. Her compassionate love and gentle manner enabled me to heal at a level of profundity I had never known before. Her gift was amazing and once again what was revealed to me was that together in community we heal, each of us connected to the Divine Source from which our gifts flow. It was God in us and through us revealing a plan that was bigger than any of us could comprehend. As a teacher, I had passed the gift of Reiki on, not only to this woman but to numerous people. Now, healers of all kinds were being drawn together to help one another unlock the burdens of life's journey. I felt blessed and privileged to have been this kind of a vehicle.

Through my own almost unbearable journeying, life's healing secrets were being revealed to me. Like Joshua, I wanted to empower others to explore their own truth and infinite possibilities for inner healing. I wanted them to honour their passages and to experience the same kind of dignity that Jesus gave to the people of His time. I was convinced now more than ever that the Jesus of history was being clothed in the ordinary garb of our day and that we, the people of God, were the ones who would be transmitting the Christ healing energy to one another.

Once again, Joshua became the Christ figure for me as I shared with him my further struggle. I told him, if possible, I wanted to be released from every buried emotion I had ever held in my body. I wanted to experience the freedom from bondage that Jesus promised if we would open our hearts wide as He did. In order to get to this point, I knew I needed to trust Joshua completely to assist me to make the body-mind connection that was necessary for my healing.

At one time, I would have been embarrassed to expose my terrible struggle to become whole, but with Joshua it was different. He radiated the love of Christ so strongly that just being in his company made one want to expose the whole truth. I told him I thought I was dealing with buried emotions. I revealed that my cheeks were ready to burst, that my teeth, head and jaws were exploding with pain. He thanked me for the information and invited me to enter the treatment with him. I totally surrendered to the plan of God asking for the healing I needed. Silently, Joshua spoke to my body to find out where the pain was coming from and the Spirit intuitively led him to ask the right question - "Did something happen to you with a group of girls at age twelve?" Instantly, my body responded and provided me with the answer. I was in grade seven at the time when the devastation occurred. After a gym class we were hoarded into the showers naked. I didn't want to go in with the other girls but was forced to do so. Even with clothes on, I had always been ashamed of my body and now, standing there in the nude I felt no bigger than a worm cringing in the dirt. All the other girls were well developed and had beautiful bodies. Mine was ugly and underdeveloped. Because of my scoliosis, my left rib cage stuck out in a peculiar way for everyone to see. From then on, shame covered me like a dirty shirt you throw in the laundry and it never does get clean.

Joshua asked me to re-enter the experience, to be there and feel what that girl of twelve felt. As I did this, Joshua said he would facilitate an opening in my head to begin the process of releasing this enormous emotion that had been stored in a place so far underground that I had forgotten it even existed. Naming the shame was one thing but inviting it to leave my body was like the inferno of a volcano, enough to blow me off the face of the earth. I remembered the volcano of St. Helen's, the blast, the devastation and then, the aftermath of some of the greatest fertility the land had ever known. Suddenly, I was filled with hope and saw my journey as no different. A few years prior to this experience I had written about shame in a poem called, "The Wisdom Of Torn Skirts."

THE WISDOM OF TORN SKIRTS

Roots in my cellar
and more roots
enough to cover me
from the shame of living here
but I am not ashamed.

Fighting for life
I've gone down under the brambles
held love like a lily
seen terror
the poisoned blackberry
cut me up like a thorn
cut me down like a tree.

I've seen death on the highway
flown into her like a blind bird.
Driving down wrong roads
in search of the right shore
for a girl to walk on
I've crossed over the bridge
called ugly
to embrace the goodness in me.

My torn skirts
have aged me considerably.

It was time, now, to connect body and mind, to integrate
my journey, to release myself from a past that had weighed me
down. For five months, Joshua, the intuitively led one, had
facilitated my healing. Somehow his heart was always led to
ask the right question my body needed to hear. Carrying God's
power in his gentle hands, my body opened under his guidance.
Buried experiences, some too deep to relate, surfaced in startling and illuminating ways. As arduous as the healing of my
memories were, it was at the same time wondrous. My body
knew and loved her journey.

Joshua was returning to Nevada but other healers with unusual gifts continued to be sent to me. The most significant
were Sheel Tangri, a specialized kinesiologist, and Anita
Horne, an Aquarian-Age healer.

Born in India and now living in Victoria, Sheel is one of
those illuminated souls emanating a Light energy that borders
on brilliant. On first meeting him, I felt instantly at home, as if
I had known him for years. His eyes were deep, dark and pene-
trating. There was something spiritual in them, something
sacred that caused me to trust him immediately. Like Joshua,
he was an extraordinary healer who had the ability to access my
body's stored memories.

I was both astonished and amazed by Sheel's treatment.
Truly, he was a man of God who touched my heart and soul and

gave me the next critical piece to the jigsaw, the information that would help me with the further unlocking of my spine. What Sheel revealed was this: at age two I had fallen and from then on my body went into a defense mode that caused the curvature in my spine to worsen. The pain of walking made sense, now - how it began as a small girl and followed me into adulthood, into the space called "crippled." I felt the nightmare would soon be over but little did I realize it would take another nightmare to integrate my healing journey.

As much as I tried to get in touch with the memory of falling, I had no recollection of it and, so, two days after my treatment, I asked God for a sign. Just before going to sleep that night, I felt like the blind daughter with mud on her eyes. Unable to piece it all together, I asked my Creator if a further healing could come through my dreams. I was awakened at quarter to five with my own screaming. I was coming out of a horrendous nightmare. Having to use the washroom, I was fully awake but lost my balance. My whole body lunged toward the concrete wall in my bedroom. First, I smashed my head on the wall and then I did a nose dive onto the floor where I hit my head in a traumatic fashion. At the same time my right arm hit my tape recorder and the fear of splitting my arm open became a reality. About forty minutes later I was in the hospital at emergency having it stitched up.

Perhaps I should have been in shock, but I wasn't. Only later in the day did the clarity come. My neck which had been stiff for years was opening and releasing and the pain in the top of my skull which had so often been diagnosed as depression was being freed up to get out of my body forever. Reliving the early trauma of this fall, was like the experience of a modern day St. Paul being knocked off her horse. I was made blind that I might see and know things to which I could not otherwise have aspired. It was a supernatural journey of meeting God incarnate in my flesh. Such inward knowledge filled me with deep and quiet joy.

Through the treatments at the Reiki support groups that

week and in the succeeding weeks, tremors of stored fear and tension continued to release through my body. If it takes a major earthquake to lead one to enlightenment, then I could say that the reliving of the fall did just that.

Along with Sheel's intervention, Anita Horne is another Spirit-led woman who needs to be acknowledged for the integral part she has played in my healing journey. Her love and support have been unconditional. Arriving at the right moment, her dedication to helping me and her special skills in the field of Bio-Mechanics and Bio-Engineering were exactly what my body needed. The severe distortion in my spine is correcting itself with Anita's help and the underground pain is being relieved as she continues to work with the ligaments, tendons and muscles in my body. Since Anita's coming, my healing has been accelerated in a significant way. In exchange for her gifts she, too, has taken all levels of the Reiki training, and is now an integral part of the Reiki healing community.

After Anita's coming, I felt that my story of healing was ready to be shared. The book was at the publisher's for a second time, almost ready to go when suddenly I was struck down by Divine Force again. It was early morning, December 13, 2000, when the dramatic event occurred. I awoke with a start. It felt as if my body were disintegrating, as if the angel of death had come unannounced into my home. Shortly afterwards, my body was in a zone called bizarre behaviour. In an unconscious state, my wild nature emerged, and I ended up in hospital with a diagnosis that finally made sense. I had undergone a grand mal seizure from too low a sodium count. In the unconscious state, my body entered what might be described as an underground wrestling match. My body was in violent spasm for a couple of days doing its "healing thing". Violent behaviour is not permissable in real life, but in a coma you can get away with anything and come out smelling like purple lilac in the spring. On the third day when I awoke from the ordeal, I felt like Jesus coming out of the tomb. In the hospital room, the only thing people saw was my nightgown, but underneath I was wearing the white dress of transformation. People weren't ready to hear of my findings and, so, I remained anonymously quiet.

In the months that followed, the revelations continued to happen. I wanted to share them but in the world of Spirit to expose something too early is to run the risk of losing the sweet taste of its essence. There were two separate events occurring, my own story and that of our Blessed Foundress who died in 1890 and who was now making her presence known. In the midst of all this, I was like a tree being watered from the inside. My branches were growing strong and sturdy and the leaves were flourishing in ways that made the Journey worthwhile. Hidden away in my lush garden, I would remain silently alert, awaiting the next clear sign that the Spirit would send. Because of my total trust and strong faith in the ways of the Almighty, my heart and soul were open and ready for anything: life, death, good news, bad news, you name it, I was ready.

HEALING IMPACT OF MUSIC

The book, now, was on hold, everything was on hold, until the next messenger came through the door. Her name was Karen Williamson, a pure soul from Sequim, Washington, who had come to take the Reiki Master workshop with me. Karen had come a month in advance to spend a week in prayer, preparing herself for the workshop. While in prayer, she received two visions that baffled her. Being somewhat confused by them, Karen, with a little reluctance, asked to share them with me. I, in turn, was astonished because Karen had no way of knowing the details of my healing Journey, no way of knowing that I had undergone birth trauma. For me, it was a further confirmation of the authenticity of what the Spirit was doing. Before leaving Queenswood, Karen was awakened in the night with a song of blessing for me. In her song, "Daughter, Be of Good Comfort", she had captured the essence of my life story.

Since the visions and the song were so integral to the unfolding of my healing passage, I asked Karen if she could record what she intuitively heard and saw. Her letter, with the song, arrived a week later.

May 12, 2001

Dear Sister Eileen

After I met with you, I went for a long walk to the beach. On the way, a vision appeared in my mind of a baby, almost lifeless, then scrunching up in fear and/or pain. This happened several times. Later I saw her as a young girl; at first she appeared to be healthy, but then something twisted her out of shape, especially her jaw.

At times I doubted the vision, as it didn't make any sense to me, but I sensed the Holy Spirit encouraging me to 'keep watching'. At one point I heard the Spirit say, "Hold the baby in the light". I experienced a sudden explosion of light, then I saw the baby sitting upright, laughing, healthy, restored. I heard the silent words, "I will do it". I wondered what all this meant, and felt I should share it with you. It was at that time that you told me you had experienced birth trauma.

In the middle of the night, I awoke and was reaching out to God in prayer. I heard some silent words being sung: "Daughter, be of good comfort; your faith has made you whole. Go in peace" (Luke 8:48). The lyrics were added: "Let your body freely dance with your soul". I knew the Lord was giving me a song for you. Later the verses began to unfold, until the song was complete.

Karen Williamson

DAUGHTER, BE OF GOOD COMFORT

Dedicated to Eileen Curteis, ssa

Based on Luke 8:48

Karen S. Williamson, lssc

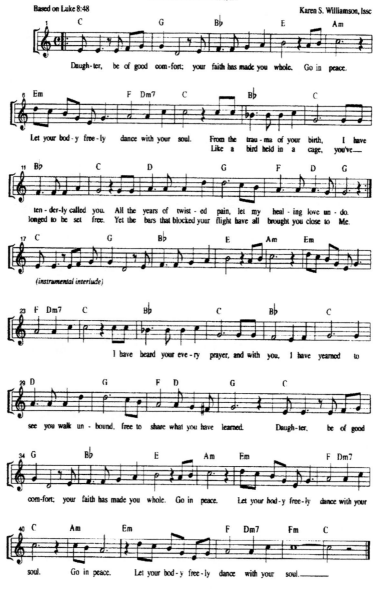

Daugh-ter, be of good com-fort; your faith has made you whole. Go in peace.

Let your bod-y free-ly dance with your soul. From the trau-ma of your birth, I have
Like a bird held in a cage, you've——

ten-der-ly called you. All the years of twist-ed pain, let my heal-ing love un-do.
longed to be set free. Yet the bars that blocked your flight have all brought you close to Me.

(instrumental interlude)

I have heard your eve-ry prayer, and with you, I have yearned to

see you walk un-bound, free to share what you have learned. Daugh-ter, be of good

com-fort; your faith has made you whole. Go in peace. Let your bod-y free-ly dance with your

soul. Go in peace. Let your bod-y free-ly dance with your soul.——

When I received the words and music to Karen's song in the mail, it was like a catalyst arriving at my door. Thirty-seven years prior I had written a number of mystical healing poems with a style very much like Karen's and I knew they were hidden away in my closet ready to be resurrected. As I pulled my poems out of the cupboard, I was inspired by God's Spirit to bring them to completion. Years ago, some people had said my poetry should be set to music but, at that time, I didn't know of anyone who could manage such a feat. When Karen's song arrived, something in me said, Karen is the composer I've been waiting for, and most definitely she was. When I phoned Karen in Sequim about the possibility, she immediately said, "Yes," and that it was an answer to prayer because she was looking for a new spiritual project to give glory to God. My own work, *Dance Of The Mystic Healer* was to be published in book form first and, then, a year later would come the full orchestration of it in musical form. Truly, the Spirit was the catalyst between us.

Today, because of Karen's contacts and mine, all the right persons are being sent, singers, musicians and others, destined to be a part of a bigger Plan. As I ponder all these unusual events, I think to myself, perhaps a Divine orchestra is ready to burst out upon the planet with God's signature written all over it.

After Karen's coming, as much as people wanted me to complete my story of healing, I knew the time was not yet. Perhaps, that's what it is to be a writer, artist and poet. You wait in dark places until the light turns green, until the next messenger comes through the door. Such was the case with Sue Hansen, a local musician and composer, hidden away in a quiet home on a hillside in Saanichton, B.C. I only learned about Sue's gifts slowly. My next book, *Soul Travel: A Roadway To Healing* was ready to go and I needed someone who could produce a CD with soft musical accompaniment as I read my work. I knew of no-one, but as providence would have it, Sue was led to me because of her interest in Reiki and she wanted to find a teacher with whom her energy could resonate.

Upon meeting me, she said I was the one. Only afterwards, did I realize Sue had all the necessary equipment at her recording music studio to produce the CD I needed. Working as a trio, Karen provided the perfect music for my meditations and Sue the subtle background music for the poems. It was truly a celebrative event where we felt the power of God working in and through us.

Just as the CD was completed, the next surprising event occurred. Karen said she had just been inspired to set the "Reiki Ideals" to music and wondered if Sue could develop and complete it in her studio. About a week later, Sue shared with me the fruit of her efforts. It was like finding a treasure in a field. I wanted to put her voice on a gold platter. What I heard was warm, soothing and professional. Her voice had the capacity to carry my message further. As well, Sue brought the wonder of Karen's composition out into the forefront where it was meant to be. We are called not to bury our talent but to stand straight and tall with what the Creator infuses. Not separate but together we form the orchestra. I showed Sue the poem of my life story that Karen had composed specially for me and, once again, Sue made the song sing in a way that was exquisite.

I knew, now, that I was called to complete my story of healing. Having these two incredible musicians enriching and supporting my story by their musical renditions was what I needed for the Voice of God to be heard more clearly. It was not just my story, but their story and all our stories being woven together.

I showed Sue a number of my poems that were interspersed throughout my book and wondered if she could lift them off the page into song, into something more ethereal than the written word. With a dubious look, she promised me nothing other than, "I'll try." A week later, she contacted me nervously saying, "I think I've massacred your poem" to which I replied, "Let me hear it." As I listened to her rendition of "Wind Daughter" my immediate response was, "You haven't massacred it! You've enhanced it, made it bloom a little more!" I continued, "So, what if you've changed a word or small phrase to accommodate your voice, you've still captured the mood and feeling and you've even made the wind whistle through her hair. If changing a word or phrase does that, then I would say, go for it." I thought to myself, Sue is an artist in her own right, dabbing a little paint here and there, making a good canvas even better. The next song she had me listen to was "Journey's Breakthrough". I instantly loved it. What she had done this time was to combine five of my smaller poems into one long song. For me, this was creative genius at its best. My heart was full. My soul was grateful. Like a song bird sent from heaven, Sue had come to play her part, to create the music and sing it well.

As Sue continued working with my poems to bring them into song, she would sometimes say, "You're cracking the whip," meaning "You're pushing me to the furthest limits of my creativity and I don't know whether I can do it." Sometimes, I felt Sue hadn't quite captured my meaning and I would make suggestions, challenging ones that sometimes seemed impossible to get to and, yet, the hand of the guiding Spirit would descend upon Sue every time. As this occurred, she would arrive at the culmination of something beautiful and, together, we would celebrate how she had been Divinely inspired. Sometimes I was reluctant to "crack the whip" and, yet, if the song didn't feel right I knew it was important to tell Sue what I felt was missing. It was hard work that required infinite patience before the song would peak, but when it did, everything in me would resonate with a "yes" that bordered on exaltation.

The last poem that I wanted to set to music was called "Straightened Tree Gone Radiant." I told Sue that it was important that this song be in the book because it told the story of how my spine had straightened through coming in contact with a community of healers. As hard as Sue tried, nothing would come. Feeling somewhat helpless and totally frustrated, Sue began listening to some music she had composed two years prior. It was an unbelievable experience. My words matched her music and instantly she was able to sing the song.

From then on, Sue, Karen and I remained open to the Spirit's guidance. Sometimes, there was a slight shift or change in words to make a song stronger or more meaningful. With the "Reiki Ideals", Sue added a second verse, capturing the essence of the Gift that had drawn us all together. Karen named the song "Just For Today", and in it lies the mystery of our healing.

You might say, "How does anyone ever end a journey like mine?" Perhaps it would be true to say one never does, and, yet, to bring my story to conclusion I shall end it this way.

A woman went on a journey to find her breakthrough, and like the vast plain of a prairie sun without end, she saw herself standing on the threshold of a new horizon. Climbing out of the closed world she was in, she could see for miles around what the future held. Free as a kite flying in the wind, she saw God mending the wing of a bird and thought it to be her. Sailing through the skies, she beheld other birds flying in similar directions - eagles, sparrows, woodpeckers - it didn't matter what size or shape they were. Each of them had been drawn together by the High One to heal and be healed. Free-spirited creatures, feathers soaring in the breeze, they would travel together from now on.

I suppose we could call this woman's journey, flight of the mystic, knowing God in the flesh and feeling again the soft energy of heaven filtering down like a warm sun after a winter day. Birds in flight, this was her journey. This is our journey.

JUST FOR TODAY

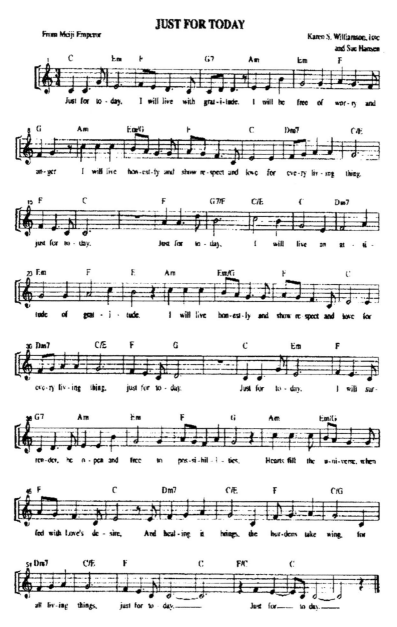

METAPHORICAL POEMS AND MEDITATIONS

Creativity is one way of actively participating in one's healing. Through art, music and poetry, I have become intimately connected with the Spirit and have been guided by that Presence throughout my life. These meditations and prose poems set to music reflect a journey that began taking me into a deeper realm of the self some thirty-five years ago. What I share here, is the fruit of that wisdom.

SPIRIT WALKER

From the beginning of time and perhaps before the beginning, I was called to live and move and have my being. The name given me was Spirit Walker. Since then, I have travelled far and learned much. In my latter years, I have moved into a home called integrity. In this quiet spot, I listen deeply for answers to come and they do come.

Just yesterday, I asked myself, "Who is this Divine healer who challenges us to follow her more closely? Where does she live? How does she act? Does she have a telephone number? And how do you get in touch with her when life loses its savour? Is she in the dog I pat or the kitten I play with? Do trees, plants, rocks and animals sing to her like I do? Is she in the air I breathe and in the flowers I smell? Is her Energy, my energy, and what about the sun, and the moon, and the stars, can I touch the glimmer of her beauty in them? Can I? And is she really a She or a He or does she go beyond gender into something more wonderful and mysterious than we can presently fathom?"

Some of us may have spent our entire lives searching for this Divine healer in the churches and we may or may not have found her. Whoever she is, wonder worker, guider of us all, in the end we must return to ourselves where the healing is needed, to let in the Light so each of us can become a cathedral of Divinity. In this way, the whole world will be lit up with Love and the face of God will never be mistaken again.

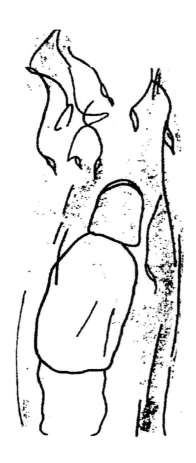

SPIRITWALKER

I believe
  in a Divine healer
  who challenges us
  to follow her more closely.
I believe in her
  and her way with us.
I believe
  if we turn our face toward her
  we'll find our darkness light
  our journey whole.
I believe
  she comes in moments
  when we least expect
  and opens doors
  that lead us to her.
I believe
  in the greatness of her Spirit
  and in the power
  of her resurrection
  to destroy all evil from us.
I believe
  and will never stop believing
  she is the Source of Love
  in our world
  and that from her
  only goodness flows.

SURRENDERED

Imagine a sky full of kites, strings dangling in the breeze. They could be people letting go of their props for the first time. Props are those things we count on to hold us up, to give us security but sometimes the prop is not the prop we thought it would be. It lets us down, disillusions us, like the educational system we thought would have the answers but didn't or the medical world not equipped to answer our kind of problems. It could be anything from abuse to a friend deserting us, which brings me to the poem "Surrendered" and the sketch of the hunch back girl who had a lesson to learn.

It all began on an eight day retreat in August, 1991, where she heard the words, "Surrender your body to me." Little did she realize that in this act of surrender her whole life would be turned around and moved in a direction the Spirit had always intended.

Her body would become her teacher and she would give it to God daily as the vessel that needed healing. She would honour her journey, the agony and ecstasy of it, and she would invite others to explore the wonder and magnitude of the gift she would bring.

Reiki had changed her life, transformed her, made her whole. From now on, she would teach others how to surrender to the healing power of Divine energy, inviting them to visit places perhaps never travelled before.

Like her, they would become explorers of a new terrain, inner astronauts travelling at lightning speeds toward God at their centre.

SURRENDERED

Not to escape life
but to plunge into it
headlong
opening myself
as it were
to an infinite number
of possibilities
choosing
not which way
I shall go
but letting the Voice
that beckons
decide it as I go.

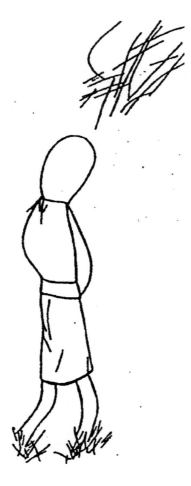

BREAKTHROUGH

Have you ever been through a breakdown? It's a scary place to be. It's like the Humpty Dumpty you learned about in grade one, only this time it's for real. You're thirty-nine and it shouldn't happen to you but it does. Everybody wants to fix you but they don't know how. The medical world tells you it's all in your head. There's nothing physically wrong with you and, so, you leave the office imagining it's all in your head. The counsellor supports this view and says, "When you get it together everything will be fine. You'll soar like a bird." Ha! Ha!

You're out on the street, now, supposedly well. The externals look good. You've learned to be assertive and nobody's going to put mud on your coat this time. You walk around with your head upright. You're not crazy after all. You do have it together but inside a voice says, "You don't have it together!" Twelve years later, I'm pretending not to limp but I do limp. The pain has overtaken my body. I run to the doctor for medication but nothing will touch it not even his arrogance. I can't sit, walk, stand, lie down. A spine crippled with pain, I tell myself, it's time Humpty listened to herself.

Leaving the doctor's office, my body thanks me. She is wiser, now. "Come," she says, "I will take you on an unplanned journey, far down, deeper than you have ever gone before. It will be filled with Divine Presence and you shall become a disciple of the inner way."

You, the reader, may say, "It's weird for a body to talk to you that way," but I can assure you, it's not. The body has so much to teach us and after travelling intimately with it these past ten years, I've come to know more about myself in this short time than in the sixty years that preceded it.

When we face our bodies honestly, we can't help but go through the door called breakthrough. The body carries its own cellular story, immense and sometimes hard to hear, but we must hear it. We need to honour its passage, to be patient and give ourselves time to heal. It takes courage to climb a mountain, maybe ten, twenty in a row, to release old hurts, wounds, scars, repressed feelings, those hidden things that may have been buried there for years, perhaps centuries. It may be the hardest work we will ever do, but we must do it. Releasing ourselves from the past, we will become free human beings, alive and creative, unleashing the full potential of our God given gifts, and with it will come an energy of Love, like fire!

JOURNEY'S BREAKTHROUGH

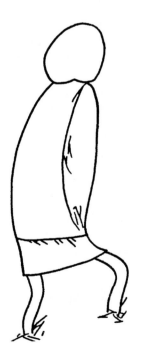

She set out
on her journey
with unchained longing
and the inspiration
that had been afforded her
to tell the people
that the breakthrough
had come.
This time
it was as if
she had been set ablaze
by the courage of newness
and with that kind of a power
she would risk
whatever was necessary
for the discovery of
her own potential
and the potential
of others.

A CALL TO REVIVAL

Canadian by birth, I sometimes wonder how I arrived on this planet, at this time, in this place. They call me, daughter of the sun, and it is true I have everything and lack for nothing. I am a Reiki practitioner, well fed and wearing the prettiest of clothes. God's love is in me and I am filled with the wonder of it. I touch others and they are blessed and they bless me. Our hands are the channels of God through which this healing flows. It would appear as if we had never struggled, as if utopia were ours. Not so!

We have come to this place, some of us fragmented, on bended knee. It was not the sunshine that led us here. Lost souls, we wear our torn shirts on the inside, each of us having fallen into one kind of a pit, or another, some of us several. We want to stand tall but in our consumer society, not to mention our religious society, we don't show our true faces to anyone for fear that shame would cover them. Thank God, we're coming out of the maze together, dishevelled, yes, but more human and whole. We're coming out of the boxes we were in. No more hiding. No more judging. No more labelling. No more ridiculing.

We're just plain people, all of us cogs in a wheel, looking at society in a new way. Oh, yes, there'll be the competitors out there, but we're not one of them. There'll be those that curse our dysfunctional families, but we'll say, "Bless them, honour them, they know not what they did." As for the churches, we have no claim on any one of them. Christian and non Christian alike, we get to hang our tapestry together. We may be small in number but who knows how the leaven will grow?

We could be in a third world country, the have and the have nots, asking the same questions. Where do the healers come from? Does it take a Mother Teresa or a Jesus Christ to fan the world with love or could it be as simple as all of us sharing our cup of water with just one thirsty soul? Who knows where the leaven will come from?

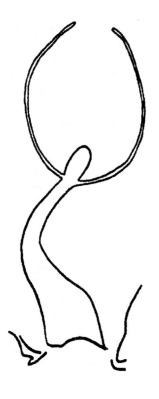

A CALL TO REVIVAL

Again and again
she would celebrate
the gratification
of it
but right now
like any daughter
of the sun
she was on the forefront
of her new world
saying
that the energy
of this warm flow
was there
for anyone
who wanted to be
inundated
by it.

VIRGIN BIRTH

Nothing. Nothing. Nothing. The place where emptiness and fullness reside, the valley I accidentally fell into when the last ounce of my existence died, the place where sweet grape and sour lemon lodge together, that place where the human soul comes home to itself in all its grandeur. Call it bliss, if you will, and celebrate it everywhere you go.

As much as my soul wanted to sing out its new found knowledge, it wouldn't happen immediately, at least, not until I had gone down the road called detour. It's a terrible, horrible, wonderful place where I found myself chugging up hill on a jalopy most people resist getting into. The pavement was hard and rough and my body, the rock, began to crumble under it. I hated this place, loathed it, spat on it, kicked it. Surely, no doctor in his right mind would have sent me here, and, yet, here was where I was meant to be. Getting in touch with my bodily rage, you could have sworn I was another Christ in the temple turning the tables of the money changers over. Yes, I had been desecrated; so many times that the fumes were toxic, but, oh, what a blessing to be rid of that which was holding me down. Just as I felt free, liberated, ready to tell the whole world about this miracle, my car suddenly skidded and I was thrown out of the vehicle, face down, flat in the mud. Was this the garden of Gethsemane Jesus spoke about? If it was, I wouldn't suggest anybody wallow in it and, yet, wallow in it I did. Everything from grief soup to shame pudding started surfacing and I was ready to let go. Oh, how I was ready! Guilt, fear, anxiety, stress, strain, everything was leaving my body. I felt ten, twenty, thirty years younger. The wrinkles were going, the muscles loosening, the spine straightening.

After ten years of persistent healing, it was a joy to behold myself and to look out at a community of healers who had journeyed with me to the place called well.

VIRGIN BIRTH

Out of a valley
of
NOTHINGNESS
she came
a woman
clothed in white
singing
a new song.

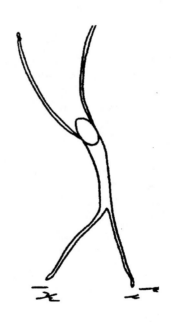

THE NEW EARTH

Pretend your body is an incubator you climb into. Others are in there with you, hatching at phenomenal speeds, but you're a slow one, premature the whole way. Grandmother earth is waiting for you. She waits and waits. You're not an ordinary chick and she knows it. A depleted body, staggering down hill, you want to be out there with the others, but it's not your turn yet.

Everything is slow, eternally slow. It's not a matter of hatching once. You're out there doing it repeatedly. One minute you think you're a chick and the next thing you know, you're an octopus, eight legs going in all directions. Didn't you know, you're too busy doing too many things? That's why people get put in incubators. They don't learn the first time round, or the second or third, and you, happen to be one of them. Think about it. It's not just incubation you're learning. A whole new way of life can develop in here.

Being cozy and warm isn't going to last forever. The egg needs to grow into a full fledged something. If you think placid, you're mistaken. You'll never get healed that way. Honesty is a better route, so why not face it, you have a wild spirit like that of a stallion, and you need to tame her. You may defend yourself by saying, "I was a little girl once, wearing an old mother hen's dress," but surely, you don't have to keep wearing it. You're a big girl, now, and you need a change of scenery. New pants, new shirt, new top, new everything.

It's time to look at your history. Get out there and start budging your body over the hill. Times have changed and there are new rules to live by, not the eight legged ones that kept you going bumpety, bump, limpity, limp. You're into a whole new way of being. Feature an octopus with an extended ninth leg. That's you at the turn of the century. It's the year two thousand and you're one of those new millennium oddities.

It's a strange passage you're into. Your heart could be do-ing cart wheels on a ferris wheel and your body feeling its way out of the dungeon. As much as you want fluidity, you can't make it happen. The body is grandmother to the soul and when one leaps, the other smiles. Healing is like that. It takes years for the repression to come and years for the repression to go. The end of it, dexterity, the time when Great Grandmother picks you up, flings you into her arms and says, "Go, now, with the wings of the earth upon you."

THE NEW EARTH

When you have been
destroyed
by the masses
you will surprise them
by your new vitality
and of your diminishment
you will say -

The blessing
of the new earth
be upon you
for do you not see
that the grace and ease
with which I move
is part
of the dexterity
of the new earth
I come from?

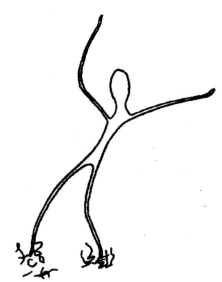

PROSE POEMS AND SKETCHES

Back in 1966, a compelling Spirit guided me to write these poems. As difficult as my life was and has been, I was charged with a strange kind of hope that to this day has never left me. As I reread the poems in 1977, I was visited by the same compelling Spirit and saw on the page beside each poem the sketch that I was meant to draw. My soul was inundated with joy, so much so, that I no longer question the deviousness by which I have been led. For one who had no art sense, I was amazed at the gift that was given. What I share here, are a small number of the poems and sketches that have been taken from my unpublished work. They tell the story of my healing simply and straightforwardly.

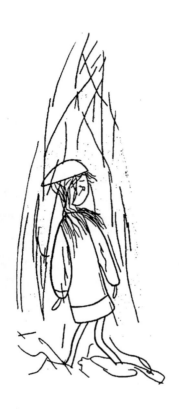

Flute Player

Your touch
invades me
like the dawn
and I run
with the flute
of a shepherd
in me.
O earth,
I say,
land, sea and sky
all burdens cease
when I bear
the wonder of you!

Released

**After long hours
of knocking
she stood
at the door
of her being
as one
purified
for the road.**

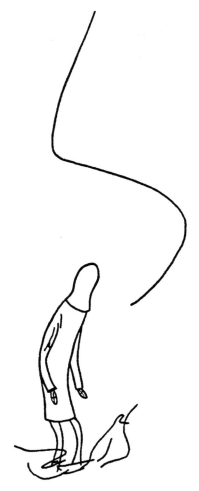

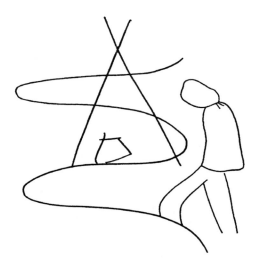

Tent Dweller

For this kind of nourishment
to happen
the heart must die
several times
before it can say
with any certainty -
I've walked past eventide
and back again
to find out life
that on the threshold of it
there lies a tent
a home
for one who had no home
though city lights
know not its name
there dwell I.

Simplicity

She did not have to repeat
the former tangle
of her life
to anyone -
she just needed
to be clothed
in the simplicity
of the remnant
that she wore
and for that
she said
nobody needed to know
the precise moment
at which the complexity
left her.

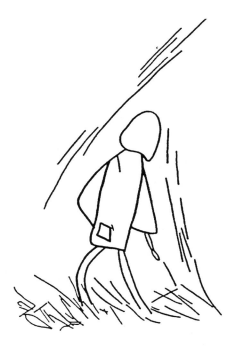

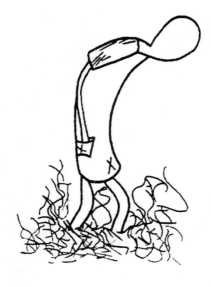

Humility

**Said the woman
who had confronted herself -
I am open
to meeting any person
on any road
at any time
for I am no longer afraid
of my weakness
which places me
below
the person I encounter
and, yet,
for all good purposes
I am on a par
with the world
as I see it.**

Resurrected
Stumbler

Once you admit
to being knocked down
you will never be ashamed
to cling to the garment
for your strength.

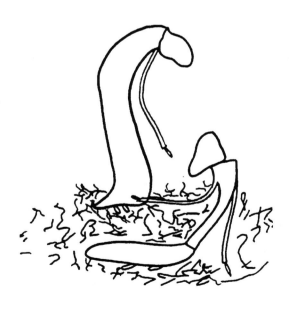

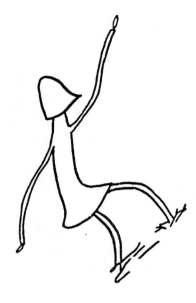

**Moments
Of Glory**

**Only the desolate
know about these things
the fog walkers
in search of Light.**

Alive With
The Seasons

She pondered quietly
how each season
could be beautiful
as the next
and to herself
she said -
Nobody has to tell me
I am alive from the inside
I just know it
and with every step I take
it's like relishing something
for the first time.

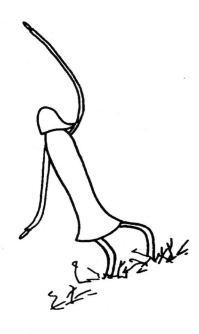

Faith Walk

Stand firm in your faith.
Let the unknown
be your guide.
Let it lead you
to the dawn
of your awakening powers.

Long
Journey

**Like all travellers
in search of wholeness
there is a force
that drives us
from the roots up.
We cannot describe it
in terms of days
months or years
we only know that
in the forest of life
we travel far
to get there.**

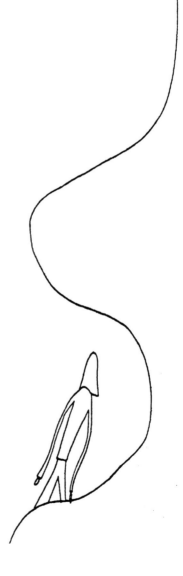

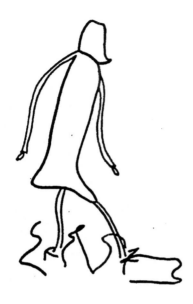

Heart Dance

I ask you
my desert Love …
If there is a Song
to be sung
then I need must be driven
to sing it !

CD CONTENT

1. **Introduction to Songs**
2. **Just For Today**
3. **Daughter, Be Of Good Comfort**
4. **Childhood Revisited and Healed**
5. **Wind Daughter**
6. **Spirit Walker**
7. **Alive With The Seasons**
8. **Journey's Breakthrough**
9. **Straightened Tree Gone Radiant**

10. **Introduction to Poetry**

11. **Self Portrait**
12. **Small's World**
13. **Lonely Stance**
14. **The Girl Called Worry**
15. **I Found My Poppies Outside The System**
16. **June Day**
17. **Magnet Woman**
18. **Even In Death Dad's Love Will Heal**
19. **Behind The Eyes Of The Blind One A Sun Shone Through**
20. **Fire Woman**
21. **Tent Dweller**
22. **The New Earth**
23. **Long Journey**

SONGS:

Performed and arranged by Sue Hansen.
'Just For Today' - Composed by Karen S. Williamson
                                    and Sue Hansen.
'Daughter Be Of Good Comfort' -
                        Composed by Karen S. Williamson.

LYRICS:

As listed above: # 4 - 9 , by Eileen Curteis,
 performed and arranged by Sue Hansen.

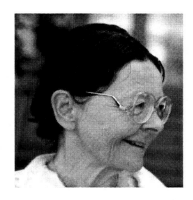

AUTOBIOGRAPHICAL NOTE

Born and raised in Victoria, British Columbia, Sister Eileen entered the Congregation of the Sisters of Saint Ann in August 1961. Sister Eileen trained in education and spent many years in this field. Over the past eleven years her path has taken a new direction, and she has been actively involved in a healing ministry at Queenswood, a retreat, growth and renewal centre in Victoria, administered by the Sisters of Saint Ann.

Sister Eileen is also the author of:

- *Risk* (The King's Men, 1975)

- *Sojourner, Know Yourself* (Sisters of Saint Ann, 1993)

- *Moving On* (Ekstasis Editions, 1997)

- *Wind Daughter* (Ekstasis Editions, 1998)

- *Dance of the Mystic Healer* (Sisters of Saint Ann, 2001)
  includes a CD on which Sister Eileen recites her poems, accompanied by Karen S. Williamson's background music.

- *Soul Travel: A Roadway to Healing* (Sisters of Saint Ann, 2002)
  includes a CD on which Sister Eileen recites her poems, accompanied by Karen S. Williamson and Sue Hansen's background music.

- *Dance of the Mystic Healer: Resurrection Songs*
  CD : Sister Eileen's Poetic Lyrics
  Music and arrangement by Karen S. Williamson

ISBN 141202165-0

9 781412 021654